THE HORSE OWNER'S
VET BOOK

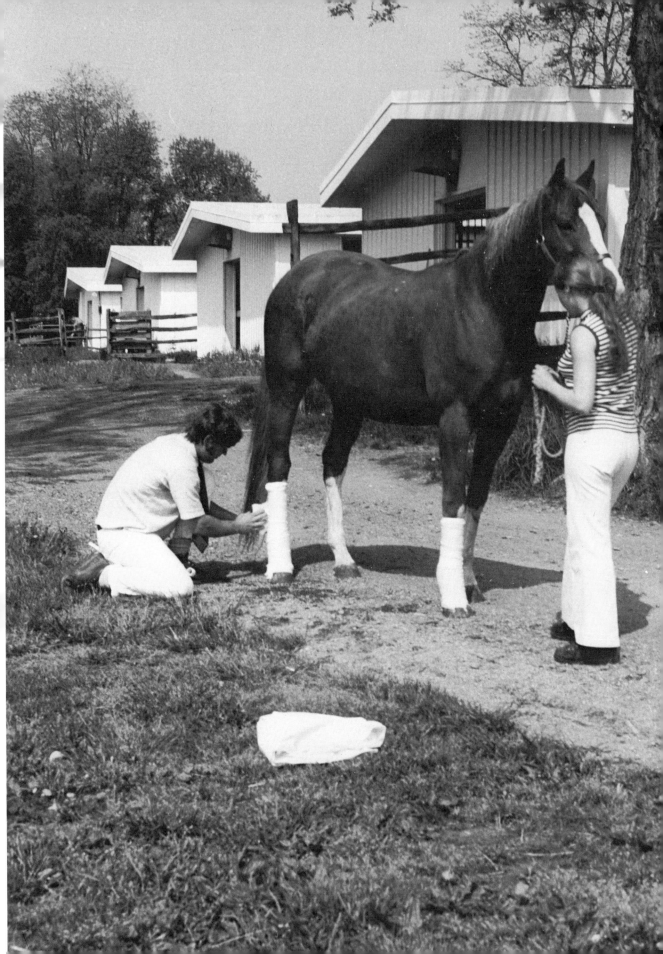

Revised and Updated Edition

THE HORSE OWNER'S VET BOOK

Recognition and Treatment of Common Horse and Pony Ailments

E. C. STRAITON

HARPER & ROW, PUBLISHERS
Cambridge, Hagerstown, Philadelphia, San Francisco,
London, Mexico City, São Paulo, Sydney

1817

U.S. Library of Congress Cataloging in Publication Data

Straiton, Edward Cornock.
    The horse owner's vet book.

    Includes index.
    1. Horses—Diseases. I. Title.
SF951.S89 1979   636.1'089   79-12266
ISBN-0-397-01344-2

*A different version of this book has been published
in England under the title* The TV Vet Horse Book.

Frontispiece photograph by Don Bender.

The following photographs are by Charles E. Ball: p. 16, "Parts of the Horse"; chapter 1, photos 1, 2, 3; chapter 2, photo 2; chapter 5, photo 7; chapter 7, photo 1; chapter 8, photo 4; chapter 10, photo 4; chapter 11, photos 2, 3, 4, 7, 8, 9; chapter 16, photos 1, 2; chapter 32, photo 3; chapter 47, photo 1. By Gary & Clark: chapter 11, photo 5.

Chapter 2, figure 1 is from drawings by Mrs. Mary L. Wakeman.

Chapter 12, figure 1 and photos 1, 2, 3, 8, 9 are from *4-H Horsemanship Program, Unit 2: Horse Science.*

Chapter 49, figures 1, 2, 3, 4 are by Dr. R. Gordon Greeley, from *The Art and Science of Horseshoeing.*

To my friend John Harvest

Contents

Index   217

Foreword

Having devoted my life to horses and riding, I have a sincere affection for all animals that enrich our days by their unflinching loyalty, that give us so much pleasure and every so often need our protection. For this reason and for the appreciation which I feel toward the author, it gives me great pleasure to write a foreword to his excellent book.

In all civilized countries nowadays friends of the animal have joined in powerful associations and obtained government support to fight cruelty to animals which may occur in our matter-of-fact times and is partly due to man's nature and more often to his ignorance. It is our noble obligation to help and protect the creature entrusted to our care. Help, however, can be given effectively only when knowledge governs the action. And knowledge, in turn, must be based on experience. In this respect, I welcome the publication of this manual.

In the sixty years of my life with horses I have witnessed with regret the great upheaval of our ways of life when the horse that was man's loyal companion through thousands of years disappeared from the army, the roads, and the farms. The army, together with the veterinary officers, had set up strict rules for the training and the care of the horse which had a decisive influence on the keeping of private riding and draft horses.

Contrary to the use of the horse for labor, his use as a riding horse has grown thanks to the increasing interest in the sport of riding in recent years. Horse lovers note with pleasure that the sport of riding has become most popular, but this fact unfortunately entails a lower standard and also a large number of often excellent horses prematurely worn out. Too many people keep horses without having the faintest knowledge about their maintenance and care. Out of ignorance, carelessness, and indifference irremediable harm is inflicted upon our loyal companion. Since in all countries there is a great shortage of riding teachers as well as grooms, qualified help in the stables is hard to come by. Many things which were taken for granted thirty years ago become problems for modern horse owners. They may face situations for which they lack the experience, and small complaints, if not recognized and treated in time, may develop into serious afflictions.

This book, therefore, fills an important gap in the field of stable management and horse care and is addressed both to the rider and to the horse owner. 11

The simple and precise explanations are clear even to the noninitiated reader who learns how to recognize the symptoms of the disease, how to apply first aid and, most important, at what moment to call for the vet.

And now a few words for the author, whose knowledge and practice of many years become obvious in every page supporting the theory of this book. Having published several books on riding which were the result of a lifelong experience, I am in the position to appreciate this particular value of a practical manual. The excellent illustrations give proof of years of patient work and represent a valuable complement to the text.

As a rider I have always considered as a good friend the vet who took care of my horses. I bear the same feeling of sincere friendship toward the author of this book, which will help us to understand and protect our loyal companion and safeguard the welfare of the horse. I am certain that my opinion will be shared by riders, breeders, and all readers who have a heart for animals and who, with me, will be grateful to the author.

Colonel Alois Podhajsky
Former Director of the Spanish Riding School, Vienna

Hofburg,
1010 Vienna

Author's Preface

Ever since I entered the veterinary profession, I have felt the need for an easily understood horse reference book, and I have always meant to produce one just as soon as I could write with absolute authority. Since only intensive or lifelong experience can give that authority, I had thought that such a book would have to wait a few years. Then a golden opportunity presented itself. Harry Robb, who had taught me as a student at Glasgow Veterinary College, retired and settled down just over thirty miles from me. Harry had all the qualifications —a long lifetime in practice crammed with intensive horse work. In fact few, if any, living veterinarians could match his equine experience.

Anyone in any profession knows that the important thing is not so much having the knowledge as knowing where to confirm it—and I had found the ideal consultant literally on my doorstep.

For several months I traveled the sixty-odd miles to and from Harry's farm twice weekly. Harry taped his memories of each condition, and we transcribed and discussed the tapes together, often grilling each other late into the night. This book is the result.

The language has been kept simple so that it can be understood by even the youngest of pony owners and riders. At the same time, the work should be equally valuable to all adult horse owners, to veterinary students, and to the many veterinarians of our time whose horse experience is extremely limited.

I wish to acknowledge not only the sterling and vital cooperation of my consultant, but also the work of Tony Boydon and Richard Perry, who are responsible for the majority of the illustrations.

Others, in the United States, have helped too—notably Charles E. Ball, writer, editor, photographer, and horseman, and Dr. R. Gordon Greeley, of the College of Veterinary Medicine at Texas A&M University.

Since completing the manuscript, I have learned with great sadness of the passing of Harry Robb. It is my wish, therefore, that this work should be a permanent and sincere memorial to his name. He was, without doubt, one of the finest veterinarians and gentlemen I have ever had the privilege of knowing.

SOME BASIC ADVICE

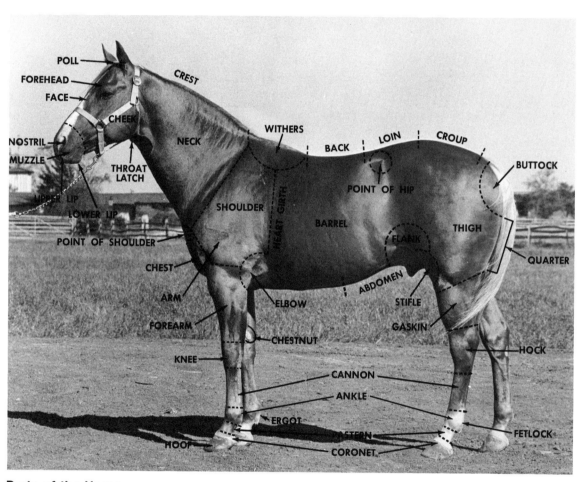

Parts of the Horse

1. Breeding

A simple knowledge of breeding is valuable to all horse owners. While raising horses is primarily a specialty for professionals in the breeding business, many amateur horsemen want to breed their favorite mare and raise a foal *(photo 1)*.

As a result, the United States horse population is rapidly increasing—from 2,955,000 in 1959 to about 8,500,000 now. (The peak was 1925, when there were 25,742,000 horses and mules.)

Choosing the Sire

The first question is, *Which stallion or sire should be used?* Regardless of breed, you naturally want a stallion with good conformation, good movement, and good temperament. One rule of thumb is to select the best possible stallion (with the best show record) that you can afford. Stud fees can range anywhere

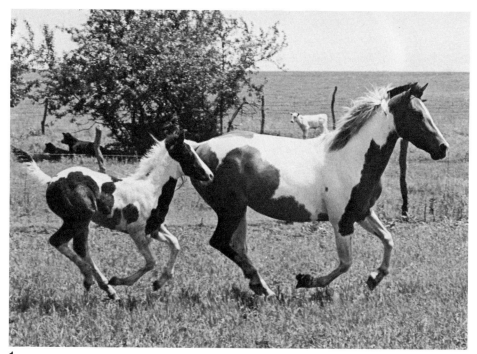

1

from $50 to $5,000. (The stallion Otoe in *photo 2* is one of the most outstanding Quarter Horse sires of his time, with a stud fee at the higher end of that scale.) For service of a good registered stallion, you might expect to pay between $500 and $2,500. Generally, the price of a racing animal starts at this point. Usually, the stud fee will be minor when compared to all your other costs in raising the foal to show age or riding age. After selecting the stallion, contact the owner and enter in contract well ahead of time for service, especially if you have selected a popular sire.

The next question is, *When should the mare be bred?* The period of gestation (time between conception and birth) is approximately eleven months. However, mares occasionally foal in ten and a half months and some take up to twelve months. So if you want a foal in January, for example, plan to breed in February.

Most breed registries count the age of horses from January 1. So owners of racehorses and show horses usually want their foals born as early in the year as possible in order to have maximum size for age. However, mares settle (conceive) more easily in the spring or early summer after the grass begins to

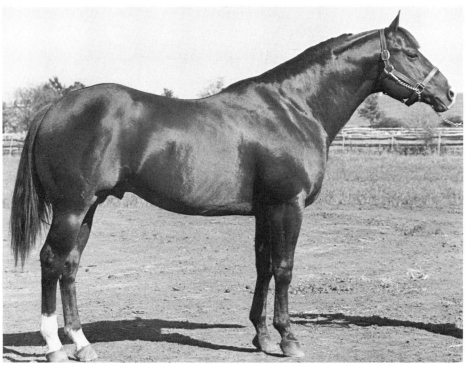

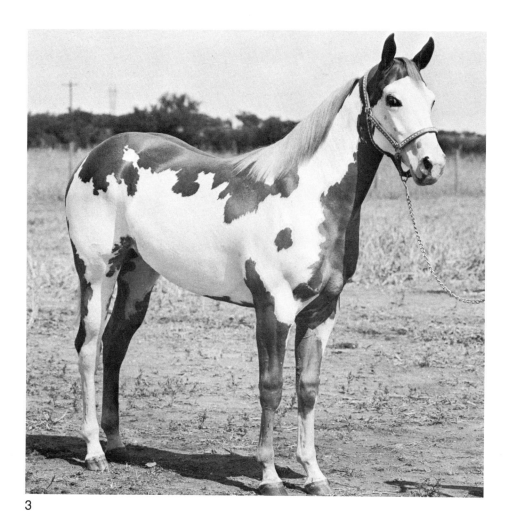

3

green up and their winter coat begins to shed. This effort to breed earlier, which is working against nature, is one reason the conception rate averages only about 66 percent in the United States. If you do not plan to show or race the young horse, you'll have much better luck by waiting until April, May, or June to breed your mare.

Conditioning the Mare

Regardless of when you wish to breed, you'll need to plan ahead. The brood mare should not be overly fat; this means that if she is in show shape, her weight should be trimmed. (The lovely Paint horse in *photo 3*, for example,   19

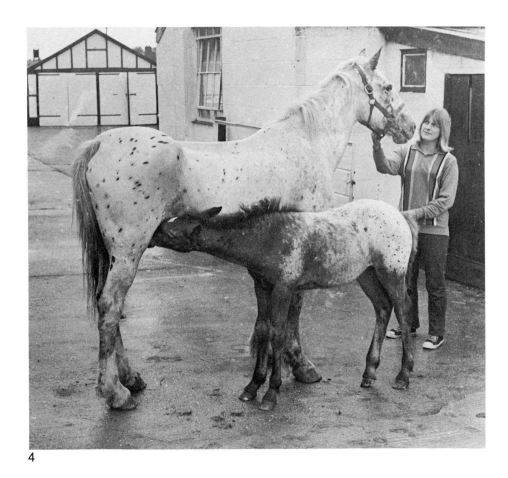
4

should lose 100 pounds or more before she is bred.) She must be in good health, however.

If she has not been bred before, you might ask your veterinarian to check her. In addition to checking her general health, the veterinarian will probably examine her reproductive organs via the rectum, making sure that her ovaries and uterus are of normal size and in normal position and also that no obstructions or irregularities, such as tumors or cysts, are present.

The Heat Period

The mare will generally cycle every three weeks and stay in heat (willing to accept the stallion) for three to seven days during the cycle. Be warned, however, that this is an average, and a great deal of *normal* variation exists.

20

The most likely time of settling her is toward the end of her heat period, although some stud managers start breeding earlier and breed two or three consecutive days.

During the heat period, within the mare, the female egg or ovum is shed from the ovary. For conception to take place, the egg has to unite with the sperm from the stallion. The sperm live only for about twenty-four hours, so if they do not meet the egg during that time the service will be a failure.

So just before breeding, your veterinarian may want to reexamine the mare as before to establish the time of ovulation. The mare may be examined as early as eighteen to twenty-one days, depending on the situation and experience of the veterinarian involved. Generally, the veterinarian will be able with a great deal of accuracy to confirm pregnancy (if it exists) at thirty to forty-five days. The rectal examination is by far the most accurate means of examination.

Rebreeding After Foaling

If you wish to rebreed the mare, she may be rebred, if she has no difficulty in foaling (no retained placenta, no laceration, no bruises, and no evidence of infection), as soon as she comes into heat after foaling. This is usually nine or ten days after birth and is called foal heat. The mare should be taken back to the stud seven days after birth to make her ready for service.

If the mare has difficulty (is torn in foaling or does not shed her afterbirth immediately), you should wait for her second heat, which is another nineteen to twenty-one days after the foal heat. Some owners prefer to breed the second heat, in any case, to allow the mare to recover completely from foaling.

When Is a Mare Too Old to Breed?

A mare is never too old to breed, whether or not she has bred before. Of course, it is much better if she starts her breeding career at an early age. The pelvis in the younger mare is more cartilaginous and relaxes more easily. Nonetheless, early service is not essential. The mare with foal in the picture *(photo 4)* is twenty-four years old.

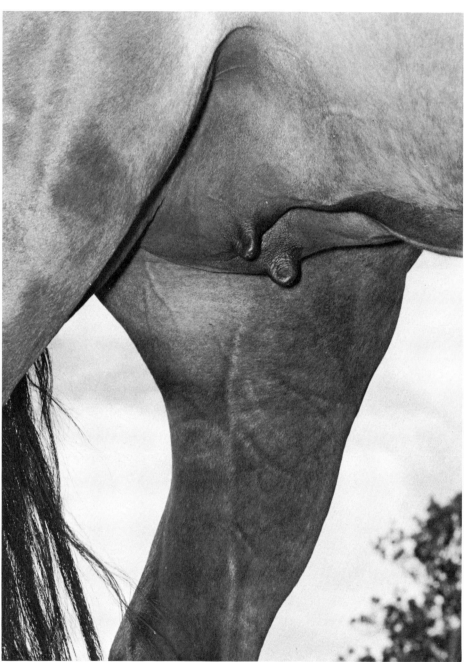

1

2. Foaling

When the foal is in the uterus, it requires nutriment and oxygen to keep it alive and growing. This is supplied by the mother, through the placenta and via the umbilical (navel) cord. Arterial oxygenated blood passes in this way to the foal's heart and is pumped through its body, then returned through the umbilical vein to be reoxygenated in the mother's lungs. The unborn foal's lungs are bypassed, and it does not breathe until after birth.

Nourishment in its simplest chemical form is also carried by the blood through the umbilical cord. And waste—urine—is disposed of by the urachus, a tube that travels part of the way through the navel cord to deposit the urine in the watery space between the two membranes that envelop the foal, like a double fluid-filled bag, and cushion the foal against damage.

When the Mare Is Going to Foal

As foaling time approaches, the udder of the mare begins to swell and a waxiness develops on the teats *(photo 1),* which may even begin to drip milk. Even with these signs, however, it is very difficult to tell exactly when the mare will foal. She doesn't like being watched during her foaling, and it will often take place at night. It can happen inside or on pasture. And because, if everything goes normally, it is over quickly (perhaps fifteen to thirty minutes), the mare's owner may sit up night after night waiting for it and then miss it by falling asleep briefly or going for a cup of coffee.

Birth

When the mare starts to foal, her uterus contracts, producing labor pains. The contractions force the foal in the watery bags against the cervix—the entrance of the uterus—causing it to open. The continued labor then moves the foal down the birth canal—the vagina—widening it to make room for the foal to pass out *(figure 1).*

If you are lucky enough to watch a foal being born, the first thing you will

23

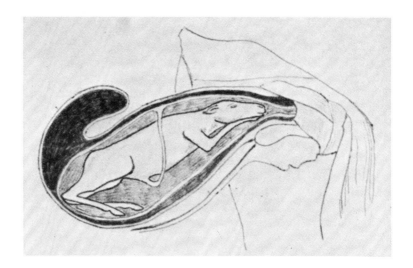

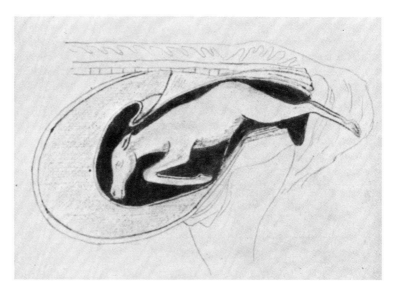

Figure 1

see appearing at the lips of the vulva will be what looks like a large balloon full of liquid. This will break and great quantities of fluid will rush out, to be followed almost immediately by the forefeet and the nose of the foal.

By the time this stage is reached, the mare's labor pains and strains are tremendously powerful and the rest of the foal soon appears. If it doesn't, call the veterinarian immediately.

24

After the Birth

When the foal is completely out, it will generally still be attached to the mother by the umbilical cord. *Do not rush to break or cut this.* Nature provides that the blood should drain from the placenta and umbilical cord into the foal.

After a certain length of time the mare will stand up or the foal will start to struggle, and the cord will stretch and break as nature intended it to do.

When the foal has been born, the mare must pass the afterbirth, or placenta —the large red or chocolate-colored organ formed early in pregnancy to supply the growing foal with all it has needed to live and develop. If this has not happened within two hours, the veterinarian must be called on for help. If the afterbirth is left inside the mare, very serious and often fatal conditions can arise such as metritis, laminitis, pneumonia, and septicemia.

The foal should be on its feet and sucking within an hour *(photo 2).* When

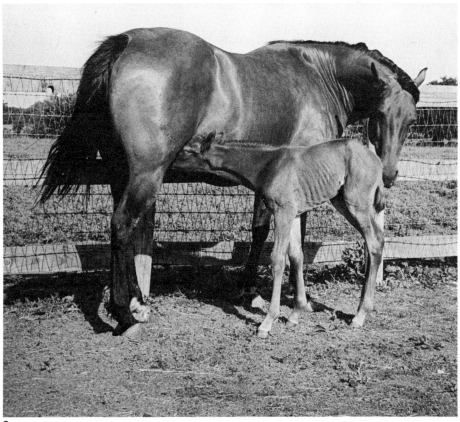

2

it attempts to get up, it will half rise and fall over several times. It is better not to assist the foal to rise. The energy expenditure is good for it, and each attempt strengthens the foal. Let it get up on its own; then you can guide it, if you like, toward the mare's udder and check that it is sucking. Your help isn't really necessary, however, as evidenced by all the foals born unattended outside that manage very well on their own.

Some people ligate (tie off) the umbilical cord and then cut it. I prefer to let it break naturally, though it is a wise precaution to dress the part of the cord left attached to the foal with an antibiotic to prevent the entrance of infection.

In addition, some veterinarians routinely give the foal (1) an enema, (2) a tetanus antitoxin shot, (3) an injection of vitamins A, D, and E, and (4) if the foal is in an unclean area, an antibiotic injection.

The mare should also be examined for tears within the birth canal, and her general overall health should be determined.

3. Problems in the Foal

Constipation, diarrhea, pervious urachus and joint ill can all present serious problems for the young foal.

Constipation

In the newborn foal's intestine there is firm chocolate-brown or almost black fecal matter. This is known as the meconium, and it is essential that it pass out as quickly as possible. During the first two or three days the mare's milk (colostrum) contains a substance called cholestron; this is a laxative designed by nature to make the bowels work and get rid of the meconium.

If within six to eight hours this meconium has not passed, it is wise to assist it by giving mineral oil and/or fecal softeners per rectum (enema) *(photo 1).*

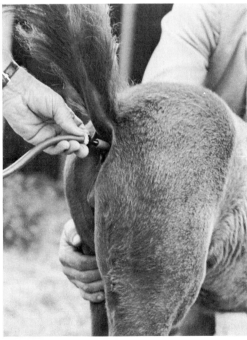

1

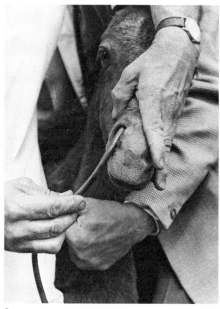

2

Such material may be given by mouth, but the enema is quicker and more efficient. This is a job for your veterinarian since, if the meconium is not passed, the foal stops sucking, develops colicky pains, and may even die.

Diarrhea

Within the first seven to ten days of life, the foal may develop diarrhea. (It generally coincides with the first heat that the mare shows.) The cause of this phenomenon has not been determined.

If the diarrhea is excessive, it is best to take the foal away from its mother for approximately twenty-four to forty-eight hours. During this period of time, the foal should usually receive a commercial mare's milk substitute. Very often it is essential that this material be given through a stomach tube *(photo 2),* since many of these foals will not take it from a bottle or a bucket. If the diarrhea is not excessive, treatment is not generally undertaken, and the foal comes out of the diarrhea spontaneously.

Chronic Scours (Diarrhea)

Later, in the event that diarrhea occurs again, as it often does, it may well be accompanied by an infection. This requires veterinary attention immediately

28

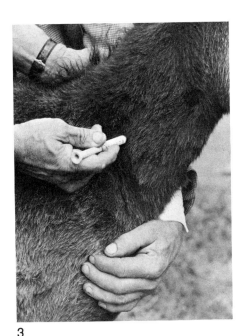

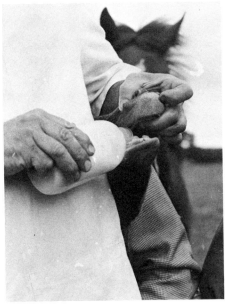

3

4

because such scours in the foal are very serious and can be terribly debilitating. Often the foal will be taken off the mare. The veterinarian may well wish to put the foal on antibiotics *(photo 3)* and in most cases will administer some antidiarrhea preparation *(photo 4)*. In the event that the foal is dehydrated, the animal will probably have to be given fluid, either orally or intravenously.

Pervious Urachus

This occurs when the urachus—the tube in the umbilical cord which took the urine away during pregnancy—fails to wither up after the foal is born and urine drops continuously from the navel.

Treatment is surgical and is usually successful. Your veterinarian should be called in as soon as possible because there is always a risk that infection will travel up the exposed urachus and set up a cystitis (inflammation of the bladder).

Joint Ill or Navel Ill

This is a pyogenic disease of foals; that is, it is caused by bacteria that form pus.

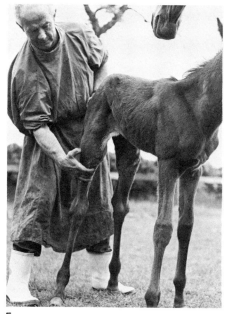

5

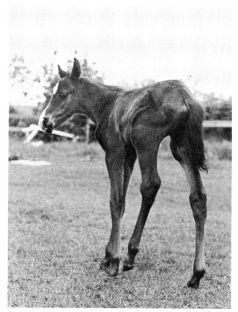

6

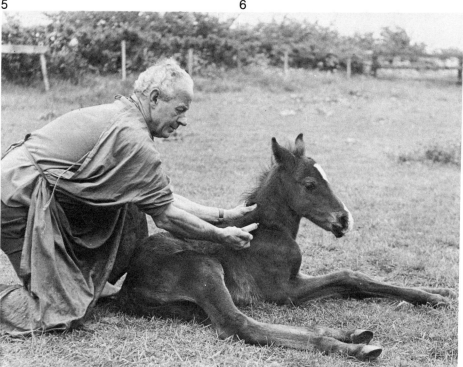

7

The bacteria gain entry into the foal through the navel or through scratches or cuts on the body. The infection may spread and ultimately involve the joints, where it starts to multiply, producing heat, pain, and swelling *(photo 5)*.

Symptoms

The first sign is lameness in one or more legs *(photo 6)*. Any lameness in the foal, no matter how slight, should be regarded as a suspect joint ill and should be reported to your veterinarian immediately.

If untreated, one or more joints will start to swell and become exceedingly painful. The pulse rate and temperature will rise, with the temperature up to 105 or 106 degrees F. Needless to say, the foal stops sucking and has great difficulty in rising, standing, or lying down. It is important to note that severe (in some cases irreparable) joint damage may take place in a short period of time.

Treatment

Successful treatment depends on immediate application, so get in touch with your veterinarian quickly. He or she may decide to inject specific and broad spectrum antibiotics *(photo 7)* and may reinforce this treatment with oral sulfa drugs. Results can be, and often are, spectacular, but remember the treatment must be started early.

Prevention

Dress the navel after birth (as described in chapter 2) with a reliable antibiotic or sulfa drug, either of which can be supplied by your veterinarian.

Good husbandry—cleanliness in the foaling box or lot—plus the conscientious dressing of the navel probably give as good if not better protection than do the vaccines.

4. Castration

Opinion varies widely on the best age to castrate a colt. Some veterinarians now castrate foals. There is no doubt that the retention of the testicles, at least for a time, helps the male horse develop in conformation and temperament. Perhaps the best way to decide when to have the operation performed is to wait until the young stallion becomes a "nuisance." He may then be a yearling, a two-year-old, or even a three-year-old.

The operation will be performed by your veterinarian but, as the owner of your prospective gelding, you will want to understand something of the technique involved.

Method of Restraint

For standing castration—the method I prefer—a twitch or a twitch plus blinkers will be needed (see chapter 8). Blinkers can be improvised by using a sweater or a towel *(photo 1)*. Needless to say, I also require a sensible assistant who is not afraid of horses to hold the head and twitch.

Injection against Tetanus

Always, as before any operation, the patient is given an injection of tetanus antitoxin, or tetanus toxoid, depending on his immune status.

The Anesthetic

Approximately one hour before beginning, I inject the colt with a heavy dose of tranquilizer. For the operation itself, a local anesthetic is injected into each testicle and into the corresponding scrotum. The twitch and blinkers are then removed, and the patient is left for fifteen to thirty minutes to allow complete anesthesia (loss of pain) of the area and the spermatic cord.

The Operation

Using a bold incision with a scalpel, the veterinarian exposes the testicles in turn. The cords are cut and crushed through by an emasculator or an emasculatome—the veterinarian may use any of several types of instrument.

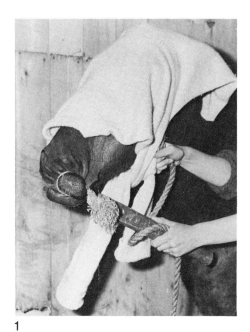

1

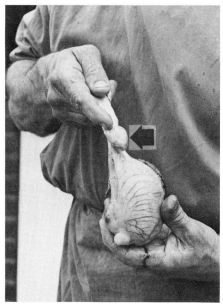

2

When the testicles have been cut free, some veterinarians—myself among them—will dress the wounds with sulfa powder. Opinions vary on the necessity for this.

Clean Cutting

The colt is cut clean when the epididymis—the small white bulb indicated here *(photo 2)*—is completely removed. When a stallion is "cut proud," the epididymides are left inside; this is often done on circus horses. The small portion of testicular tissue left gives the horse a boldness and a carriage which geldings often lack.

No aftercare should be necessary beyond making sure that the animal gets regular exercise. There are no stitches to be removed. Swelling of the area is inevitable, but there is no cause for concern unless the patient goes off his feed. If that happens, send for your veterinarian immediately.

The Ridgling (Rig)

A "rig" is a male horse which has retained one testicle in his abdomen or inguinal canal—the channel that runs from the scrotum to the inside of the   33 abdomen. He behaves like a stallion and is a real nuisance, especially when mares are present.

Diagnosis and Treatment

This is very much a matter for your veterinarian. He or she will examine the animal in a number of ways to confirm that only one testicle has been removed. The existence of only one scar on the scrotum does not necessarily mean this, since an alternative castration technique used by some veterinarians involves just a single incision. Inguinal and rectal exploration may turn up the retained testicle. If not, there are a number of procedures that can be undertaken to locate and remove it. One way is to open into the abdomen through the flank *(photo 3),* but there are several other simpler procedures as well.

However it's done, it's well worth it as most ridglings overproduce testosterone (male hormone) and can be very difficult to handle.

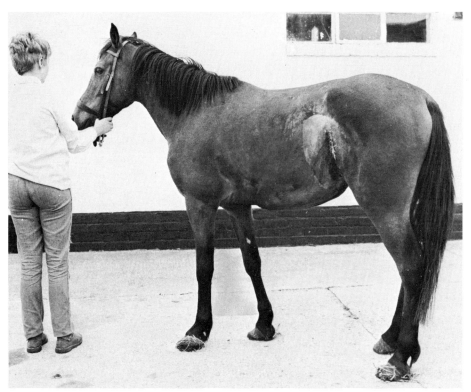

5. Feeding

Nothing is more important for the health of your horse than what he eats. In nature, the horse feeds entirely on grass and herbs plus a little earth from which he obtains certain minerals essential to his well-being.

This is sufficient for a horse running wild or during a summer period when he is doing no work. During the winter, however, and also all the year round when in work, a horse requires some additive or extra feed.

Three standard feedingstuffs for horses are hay, oats, and bran, and the quantities to be fed will depend on the amount of work the horse is expected to do. Other ingredients are usually included in commercial feeds and are very good. These include corn, grain sorghum, wheat, barley, and cottonseed or linseed or soybean meal, plus vitamins and minerals to balance the ration.

One important point to remember is that a horse's stomach is remarkably small in proportion to his size—very much smaller than, for example, a cow's stomach. If you watch a horse on pasture, you will see that he is nibbling away most of the time, resting only for short periods. He does this on through the night. Frequent eating of small amounts is a basic requirement for good nutrition.

Hay

You can make hay available more or less all the time, but *it must be good-quality hay.* Moldy or otherwise damaged hay can cause a great deal of trouble. Unless very hungry, a horse will not eat bad hay. There is no better judge of the quality of hay than a horse.

Hay can be fed in three ways: by just throwing it in the corner of the box stall *(photo 1),* in hayracks *(photo 2),* or in hay nets *(photo 3).*

If hay nets are used, they must be placed very high because they become longer as they empty and the horse, in pawing at them, may get a leg caught in the net with disastrous consequences. What kind of hay is best? Alfalfa is generally preferred by experienced horsemen, because it contains more protein, minerals, and vitamins. But there are other good hays, such as timothy, legume hay, prairie hay, and coastal Bermuda.

35

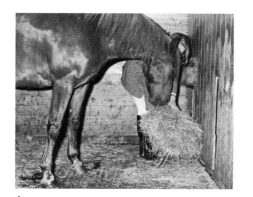

1

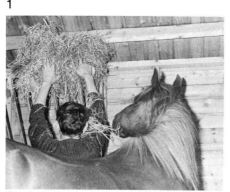

2

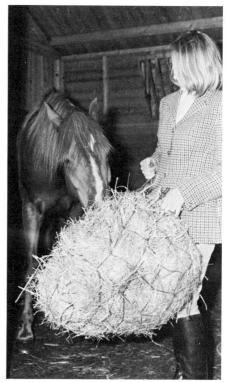

3

Oats

Before being fed to horses, oats should be rolled or bruised *(photo 4)*. Whole oats can be fed, but many of them will pass through the bowel without being digested. Other grains should also be coarsely ground or rolled.

Bran

Wheat bran, which serves as a laxative and is especially good for horses, should never be fed dry if fed alone. The horse may make the dry bran into a ball, and this can block his esophagus, causing "choke." The bran can be fed either damp or mixed with other ingredients *(photo 5)*. Even when fed with oats, bran should be dampened.

Manufacturers are now supplying horse pellets or cubes *(photo 6),* which are made from a mixture of hay, oats, bran, and other ingredients, all pressed into each cube. It is a very easy way to feed, eliminates the storage of hay, and is quite satisfactory. However, it is more expensive.

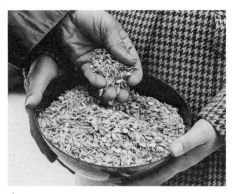

4

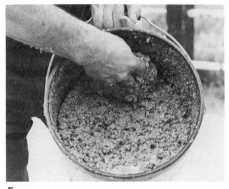

5

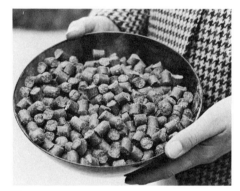

6

Times of Feeding

Feeding should be done two or three times a day, stretching the day out as long as possible from early morning until late at night. During the night, leave plenty of hay with the horse so that his stomach never becomes completely empty. In this way you simulate nature and allow the horse to live a more normal life.

Amounts to Be Fed

It's impossible to lay down hard-and-fast rules for the amounts to be fed, because different horses require different quantities to do the same work and stay in the same condition. If you are an experienced horseman, you can usually look at the horse and tell whether his feed is adequate.

If you are a beginning horseman, here are some guidelines for daily feeding:

For a horse in a stall doing only light work, allow about ½ pound of grain

37

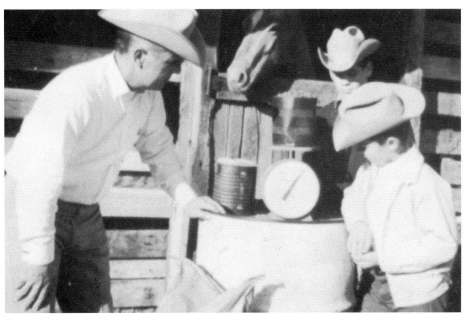

7

and 1½ pounds of hay per day per 100 pounds of body weight, plus 1 pound of protein supplement.

For medium work, feed 1 pound of grain and 1 to 1¼ pounds of hay per day per 100 pounds of body weight, plus 1 pound of protein supplement.

For heavy work, up the amount of grain to 1¼ to 1½ pounds and feed 1 pound of hay per day per 100 pounds of body weight, plus 1 pound of protein supplement.

So the average thousand-pound horse doing medium work should get about 9 pounds of grain, 10 to 12 pounds of hay, and 1 pound of protein supplement a day. Also, your horse should never be without salt, preferably loose salt fed free choice.

Most horsemen think in terms of gallons or quarts rather than pounds, so you should weigh your feed occasionally *(photo 7)*. Generally, a quart of oats weighs about 1 pound, a quart of barley 1½ pounds, and a quart of shelled corn 1¾ pounds. A bale of hay usually weighs 45 to 50 pounds.

Water

Without doubt, the most important feed of all is water, since about 50 percent of the body weight is liquid or moisture which must be replenished almost continuously. Fresh, clean water should be with the horse *constantly day and night* so that he can drink as and when he likes.

The water *must be clean and fresh*—not the bucket of "liquid manure" one frequently sees; therefore, the bucket should be cleaned daily.

Winter Keep

Many horse owners, both adults and youngsters, are full of enthusiasm during the summer while the shows and parades and trail rides are on. When winter comes, however, the horse is frequently turned out into a field without feed or shelter and forgotten. This practice indicates a cruel lack of concern for the horse or pony's welfare.

For shelter, a box stall with a half door is the ideal, though satisfactory cover can be provided by improvising any old farm building. In the southern part of the United States, a horse can get by without shelter, *if he is well fed.*

Two other important points. During the winter, even though the horse is turned out, his feet require regular attention. Every six weeks or so, just as in the summer, the farrier will have to be called in.

Finally, water—you must keep checking the drinking water. If there is a frost, the water supply may freeze over and the ice will have to be broken. Keep plenty of fresh water available at all times, summer and winter.

6. Immunization

The best treatment for any disease is prevention. So to keep their horses normal and healthy, many owners have their veterinarians routinely immunize for the more common diseases. This varies by areas, but you and your veterinarian will probably want to consider the following immunization program:

1. For *encephalomyelitis,* Eastern and Western strains, two injections each spring or summer, seven to fourteen days apart, for horses of all ages (see chapter 16).

2. For *Venezuelan equine encephalomyelitis* (VEE), one injection during the spring or summer (see chapter 16).

3. For *equine influenza,* two injections the first year, four to eight weeks apart, followed by a booster shot each year thereafter (see chapter 29).

4. For *tetanus,* or *lockjaw,* two injections the first year, four to eight weeks apart, followed by a booster shot yearly thereafter (see chapter 15).

5. For *strangles,* or *distemper,* three weekly injections the first year, followed by an annual booster until the horse is five years old. Opinion varies widely on the advisability of these injections. Many veterinarians do not consider them effective enough to warrant the risk of vaccination reactions, even sloughs, that sometimes result (see chapter 27).

6. For *rhinopneumonitis,* a generally mild respiratory disease in young horses that is capable of causing abortion in mares, or neonatal death, two injections of the vaccine, four weeks apart, followed by a booster each year. The efficacy of the vaccine in the prevention of abortion is at this time questionable. There certainly is evidence to indicate, however, that it is successful in checking the respiratory disease.

To simplify the immunization program, many owners simply ask their veterinarian to give their horses immunization shots in the spring and in the fall, without specifying which ones. After consultation with your veterinarian, you'll probably find this quite adequate.

7. Temperature, Respiration, and Pulse

To recognize symptoms of trouble, you need to know what is normal for your horse when all is well. His general appearance, his way of moving, his attitude, and his temperament can tell you a lot. But it is important to know how to test his temperature, respiration rate, and pulse rate. And when you suspect illness and call your veterinarian, it's useful if you can supply this information.

Temperature

The normal temperature of a horse is 99 to 100 degrees F. A slight variation doesn't necessarily mean disease or sickness. Sex, age, time of day, season, climatic temperature, mating, and temperament can cause the temperature to rise or fall slightly.

Some horse owners attempt to determine temperature by feeling the horse's nose, ears, or legs, or by placing a hand in the horse's mouth. But these methods are quite crude and totally inaccurate. The only accurate way to determine a horse's temperature is with a rectal thermometer *(photo 1),* which you can purchase from your veterinarian or a livestock supply store. Be sure to ask for a *maximum registering rectal thermometer* of heavy construction.

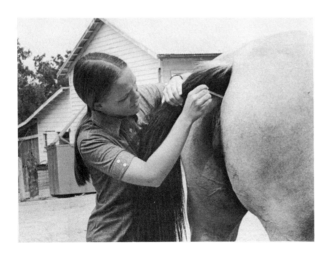

To check the patient's temperature, first shake the mercury down. Then moisten or lubricate the bulb with Vaseline or a similar jelly and place it full length into the rectum. Leave the thermometer in place at least four or five minutes, then withdraw it, clean it, and read it. It is best to attach approximately 24 inches of string to the thermometer and secure it to the tail with a clip.

Respiration Rate

The respiration rate is how often the horse draws air into the lungs (inspiration) and expels it from the lungs (expiration). Most people refer to this as inhaling and exhaling.

The normal rate is 8 to 16 per minute, if the horse is calm and standing. Of course, this increases with exercise, excitement, or stress. At the end of a race, for example, a horse may have a respiration rate of 30 to 40 and still be normal.

One good way to check the respiration rate is to stand off and observe the in-and-out motion of the ribs, timing it with the second hand on your watch. Another is to place your hand on the rib cage or flank and feel the movement each time the horse breathes.

Pulse Rate

The pulse is an intermittent wave in an artery, caused by the heart's pumping blood through the artery. The normal pulse rate for a horse is 28 to 40 per minute. Like the respiration rate, this will increase with exercise, excitement, or stress. So after running, the pulse rate may accelerate to 80 or 100 or more and still be normal. But 80 to 100 without exercise or excitement is cause for concern.

Where to take the pulse? One convenient place is the artery that runs around the inner side of your horse's jaw *(photo 2)*. Other arteries that are close enough to the skin to be felt are located on the inside of the knee of the foreleg and at the back of the fetlock joint.

When examining a horse, always check the temperature, respiration rate, and pulse rate first, before the animal gets excited, as excitement may well increase these rates.

42

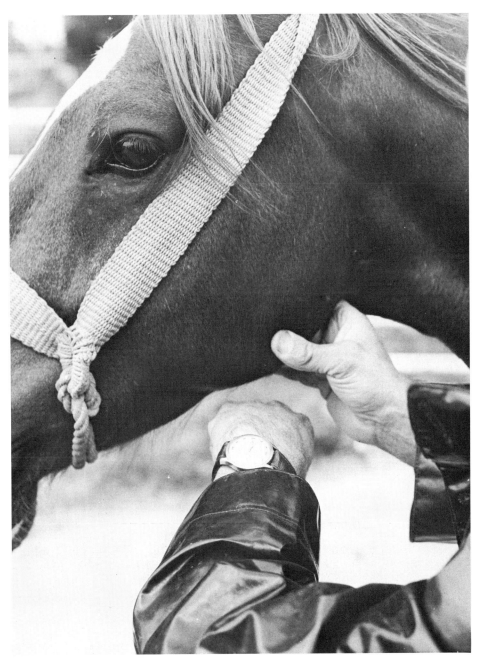

2

8. Simple Methods of Restraint

Horses and ponies are not unlike children—they like their own way and usually misbehave if they are allowed to get away with it. This can be an embarrassing nuisance, especially if you have to examine, clip, or treat them.

There are four simple methods of restraint which, used singly or together, usually allow the satisfactory handling of any horse.

Lifting a Front Foot

Obviously, the horse standing on three legs is less likely to kick or prance about *(photo 1).*

Holding the Tail

This is especially useful during the examination of a hind leg. The horse will rarely kick if the tail is held firmly downward *(photo 2),* upward, or to one side.

Applying a Twitch

As a rule, use of a twitch *(photos 3* and *4* show two kinds of twitches) is necessary only when slight pain, such as a hypodermic injection, has to be

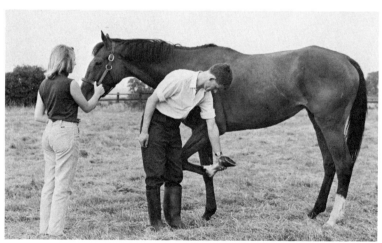

1

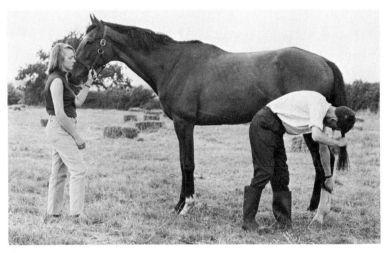

2

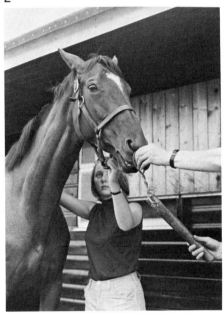

3

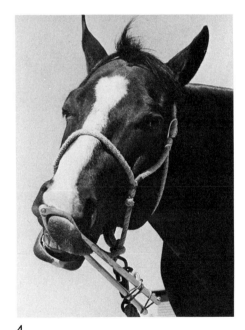

4

administered, or if the horse hasn't been handled much. The muzzle is particularly sensitive, and pressure there distracts the horse's attention from interference elsewhere. The twitch can also be applied around the base of an ear, where it works equally well. Be aware that the twitch is a painful distraction and occasionally the horse will react violently, so it behooves the handler to be alert.

45

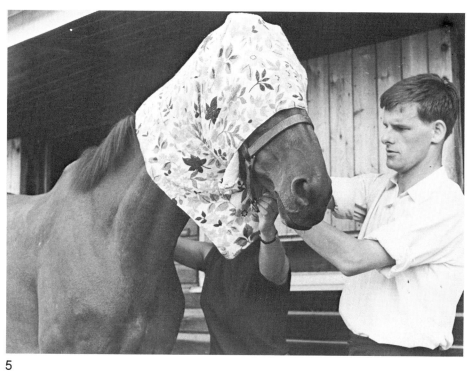

5

Blindfolding

In my experience this is one of the most valuable of all the methods of restraint, especially if the animal has to be handled in an open field. Any improvised blindfold can be used, such as a towel *(photo 5),* a sweater, a coat, or a sack. A combination of the blindfold and the twitch will usually allow the satisfactory handling of even the most fractious of colts.

Blindfolding is also useful when loading a nervous animal into a horse trailer.

46

9. Wounds

Wounds are classified in three categories: (1) incised wounds—cuts made either by the surgeon's knife or by sharp tin or sharp glass, (2) lacerations—tears such as those caused by barbed wire *(photos 1* and *2),* and (3) punctures—typically caused by a stake or a thorn or by a picked-up nail.

In incised wounds, the blood vessels—either arteries or veins or both—may be cut. The resulting hemorrhage may be severe, depending on the size and location of the vessel or vessels.

In tears, the vessels are pulled and extended and there may be little or no bleeding. This is because the walls of the veins and arteries are elastic, and, when pulled, the ends recoil within themselves and form a natural barrier.

The same usually holds true for puncture wounds, though if the puncture is directly through a large vessel the resulting hemorrhage can be severe.

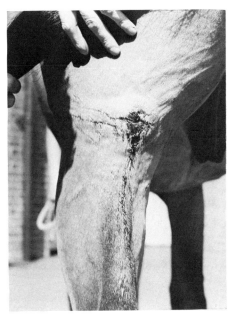 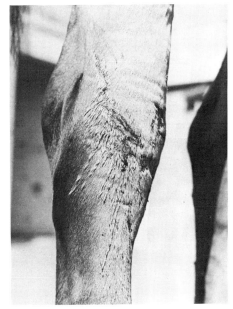

1   2

First Aid Supplies

The mistake made by most horse owners is to stock up with an excessive quantity and variety of first aid remedies, with the result that in an emergency they waste valuable time wondering which to use.

The ideal is to keep handy a comparatively small box containing:

1. Bland antiseptic soap, 8 ounces. If in any doubt about which to buy, ask your veterinarian to supply it.

2. Surgical gauze, 1 roll 3 or 4 inches wide.

3. Sterile cotton, 1-pound roll.

4. Gauze bandages, 6 large—ideally 3 to 4 inches square; anything smaller is impractical.

5. Sulfonamide or furazolidone, 4 ounces.

All the items on this list may be purchased at your drugstore or from your veterinarian.

Your first aid kit should also contain the thermometer you keep for checking your horse's temperature.

Bleeding

If a wound of any of the three categories is bleeding profusely, the first thing to do is to stop the flow. Hemorrhage (which is simply another word for bleeding) can be of two types: *venous,* from a vein or veins; and *arterial,* from one or more arteries.

Arterial bleeding is more dangerous than venous, and it is easy to distinguish between the two.

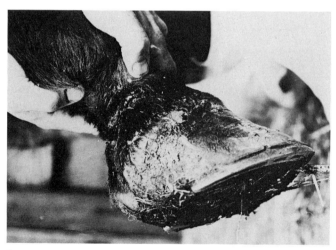

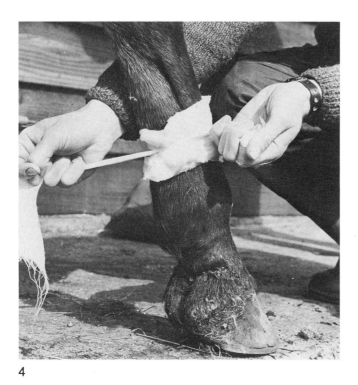

4

In venous bleeding the blood "oozes" or "flows" *(photo 3)*. In arterial bleeding the blood "spurts out" in time with the heartbeats which are forcing the blood through the arteries.

Treatment

In general, bleeding is controlled by simple pressure.

Horses' legs are particularly vulnerable to arterial damage because the arteries are comparatively near the surface. If a leg is hurt and the blood is spurting, a tourniquet should be applied immediately. This can be done by placing a pad on the course of the artery *above* the cut and covering it over with a really tight bandage *(photo 4)*. The tightness required can be judged by the pressure needed to stop the bleeding, but never leave the tourniquet on for more than fifteen minutes at one time. Why? Because, with the tourniquet pressing on the artery, the blood supply is stopped to all parts of the limb below the tourniquet. Continued pressure would lead to blood-starved tissues and subsequent tissue death.

Having applied the first aid, send for your veterinarian immediately. The first quarter-hour period the tourniquet is on probably will not give time for

49

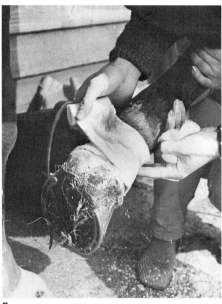

5

the veterinarian to get there. If not, release the tourniquet for *one minute,* then reapply slightly higher up or lower down.

The veterinarian will probably pick up the damaged artery with artery forceps and ligate it (tie it off). If this has to be done, the smaller arteries in the area enlarge to make up or compensate for the artery that has been lost. This phenomenon is called the development of collateral circulation.

If the hemorrhage is venous, only minimal pressure is required to control it. This pressure can be applied directly by covering the wound with a thick wad of gauze-covered cotton—making what is called a compress—and bandaging over it *(photo 5)*.

Nature plays a large part in control of bleeding by clotting the blood. In veins these clots quickly seal off the damage, but in arteries the powerful pressure of the pumped arterial blood keeps blowing out the clots.

The golden rule, therefore, is: with all bleeding—from any part of the body —apply first aid control, then send for your veterinarian immediately.

Care of the Wound

When bleeding is under control, wounds should be *washed thoroughly* with warm water containing a bland or nonirritant antiseptic; sterile cotton or a clean cloth will help remove any surface contamination. (In the case of an

50

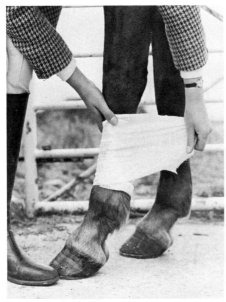

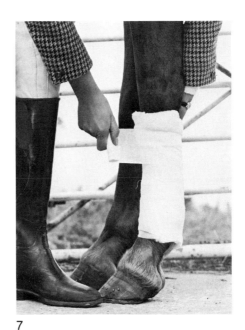

6   7

arterial wound, if the hemorrhaging has been stopped do not disturb the wound by washing but wait for the veterinarian to come.)

Never use iodine or any of the other old-fashioned irritant antiseptics; they all damage the tissues and retard healing. There are many nonirritant antiseptics on the market, most or all of which will destroy the bacteria without damaging the tissues, and your first aid kit should already have the one your veterinarian has recommended.

A sulfonamide or antibiotic dressing is an efficient aid to healing without infection, and this must be prescribed by the veterinarian, either as a staple of your first aid kit or for the specific wound occurrence. Apply after washing the wound with the antiseptic solution.

Leg wounds—the most frequent occurrences—should be bandaged as shown in *photos 6* and *7.* The method of bandaging is to cover the wound with gauze, place a layer of cotton completely around the leg, and wrap with bandage to hold it all in place. Then wait for the veterinarian.

When the Veterinarian Comes

Professional attention is important to the care of all wounds. Incised wounds will have to be stitched *(photo 8).* Tears should also be stitched if the edges can be brought together *(photo 9).* If you have already dressed and   51

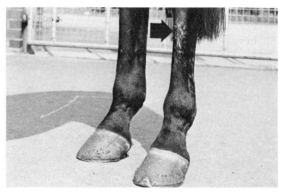

8

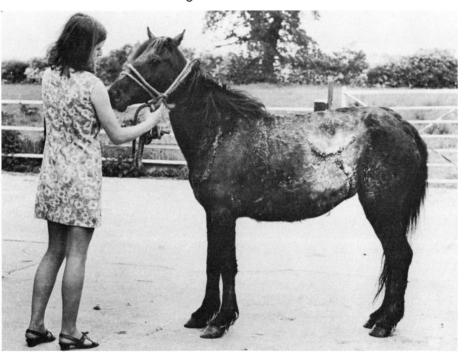

9

bandaged the wound, the veterinarian will probably want to reinforce the dressing. And it is imperative in the case of punctures that he or she inject against tetanus—with a booster shot if the horse has already been immunized. Punctures are the most dangerous in this respect, but I also recommend tetanus protection in the case of lacerations and cuts. It is wise insurance against the loss of the horse.

52

10. Self-damaging Horse Faults

Damage to the horse may be self-inflicted both by faults in conformation and by stable vices. In all cases they require the owner's attention.

Conformation Faults

Brushing

Brushing is hitting the inside of a fetlock with the opposite hoof or shoe. It frequently happens in horses with narrow chests and in those that do not move squarely but prefer to "swing a leg" or "wing in."

What to Do About It

Brushing boots, which provide a pad over the fetlock, can be used *(photo 1)*. While the brushing boot will prevent damage to the leg, it does nothing to solve or prevent the problem.

Generally such horses require little more than balancing the feet so that both heels contact the ground squarely. Further, the blacksmith should encourage the horse to break over the center of the toe. In instances where the conformation is grossly out of balance, this may be a difficult chore.

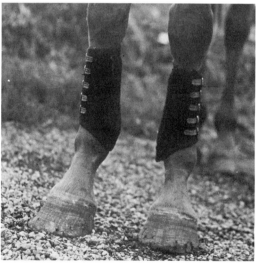

1

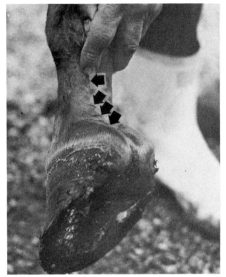
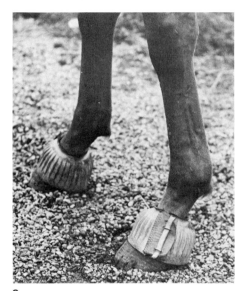

2   3

Overreaching

An overreach almost invariably occurs during jumping or galloping. The hind-foot shoe catches the back of the pastern *(photo 2)* or the bulb of the heel of the forefoot and cuts it *downward.* This cut may be slight—a graze—or it may be a deep cut involving most of the bulb of the heel.

Heavy going obviously can predispose to overreaching, since the horse may have difficulty in pulling his forelegs out of the mud before the hind feet come forward.

Treatment

An overreach wound must have prompt and skilled attention because the downward cut produces a pocket without drainage, where dirt and infection can quickly gather.

Prevention

Shorten the toes of the hind feet and shoe with light plates. Overreach boots, or bell boots *(photo 3),* should be worn, especially when jumping.

Speedy Cutting

Speedy cutting rarely happens in riding horses. It is most likely to occur in horses with a high action, like trotting ponies. In many ways it is similar to brushing, but in speedy cutting the part struck is either halfway up the inside of the cannon bone or the inside of the knee.

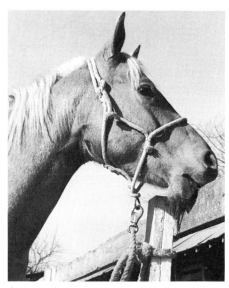

4

Prevention

Similar to that recommended for brushing, with special attention being paid to the feet and shoes.

In the attempted correction of these conformation faults, a good farrier is worth his weight in gold.

Stable Vices

Stable vices are the result of idleness. They develop in horses kept far too long in the box without exercise and are caused by boredom. They can occur at any age but are seen more in older horses simply because they do less work.

Windsucking and Cribbing (Crib-Biting)

A horse can windsuck without cribbing, or vice versa, but he often cribs in order to windsuck.

Windsucking is drawing the air into the mouth and then forcing it down the gullet into the stomach. When doing this, many horses catch onto the manger, the door, or any spar *(photo 4)*. Many bored horses will just bite or gnaw on wood. While this is not necessarily windsucking, it often leads to it.

Having drawn the air into his mouth, the windsucker then generally arches his neck quickly as he swallows the air.

Eventually a persistent offender becomes expert and can windsuck without cribbing.

What Effect Does It Have?

Windsucking may upset the stomach and lead to indigestion, which becomes chronic. Not only does the horse's general condition deteriorate, but he is more likely to develop flatulent colic.

How to Spot a Windsucker and Cribber

The teeth are unnaturally worn *(photo 5)*. If you suspect unnatural wear, observe the horse patiently and you will see or hear him at it.

Treatment

In many cases treatment is useless, but it is always worth trying.

First of all, get the horse into regular work so that when he gets back to his stall he is tired and not bored.

Remove everything and anything on which he can bite—manger, spars, etc.—and if you can't remove them, soak them in creosote. Keep both halves of the door closed so that there is no exposed edge.

Another treatment that is often effective makes use of a strap which is fitted around the neck just behind the ears and passed around the back of the jaw. This strap is as illustrated *(photo 6),* or it may be threaded through a heart-shaped piece of doubled very stiff leather. The point of the heart fits in between the angles of the lower jaw *(photo 7)*. When the horse arches his neck

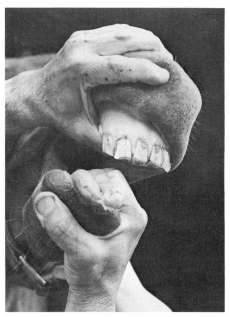

5

to swallow the wind, the point of the heart jabs him and forces him to put his head forward and let the wind out of his mouth.

Occasionally, with bad cases, a piece of metal, like a steel spring, can be fitted to the point of the leather heart device.

Some horses quickly learn to maneuver the heart out of position. When this happens, put a halter on and tie the strap in position with pieces of string or a shoelace. Installing a steel (not glass) mirror will often provide entertainment for the bored horse.

Obviously, any success in treatment will be slow, and the results will largely depend on how long the horse has been windsucking. With persistence and luck, even some of the chronic cases can be cured, but there is certainly no guarantee.

Prevention

Keep the horse or pony in regular work and soak with creosote all potential biting edges within the box stall. The creosoting should be repeated every six months.

Just one last word: Windsucking and cribbing constitute a definite unsoundness, and a suspect case should never be purchased without careful veterinary examination.

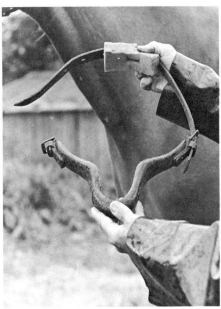 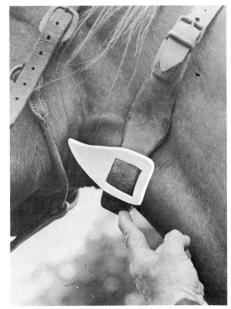

6   7

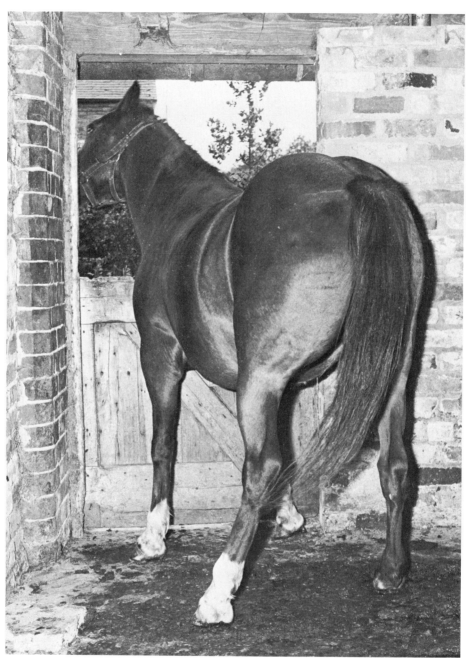

8

Weaving

Weaving is another stable vice resulting from boredom and, again, an unsoundness.

Symptoms

A weaver stands rocking from one forefoot onto the other and will often continue to do so for long periods. He will then walk around the box stall and start again.

Weaving occurs particularly in a stall with a half door that opens out into a yard. The horse will stand looking out over the door, rocking to and fro *(photo 8)*. In fact, frequently the floor will be worn in two hollows close to the door.

What Adverse Effects Does It Have?

Weaving makes the horse tired and less capable of hard work, and excessive and abnormal shoe or hoof wear may take place.

Treatment

Avoid boredom by keeping the horse or pony in regular hard work, so that when he comes back to the box he is too tired to do anything but sleep. Keep the top half of the stall door closed.

If possible, turn him out to grass. Even a bad case will rarely, if ever, weave at grass.

Prevention

If the horse is not in regular hard work, he should be kept at grass or in a paddock.

11. Saddle and Girth Sores

It is important to know the causes of saddle and girth sores, since they can usually be prevented.

Saddle Sores

Saddle sores are sores that appear on the back under the saddle *(photo 1)*. They have various causes, almost all of them controllable by the horse's owner. They basically represent local excessive friction. They may occur in varying degrees from superficial hair loss to deep, painful sores.

A well-fitting saddle *(photo 2)* must be the correct length for the size of the horse. A reputable saddler is the best person to advise on this.

The seat of the saddle should fit smoothly and evenly on the back.

The pommel, the arch at the front, must be high and well clear of the withers *(photo 3)*.

The cannel or tunnel running from the front to the back must be clear, permitting the passage of air and never at any time exerting pressure on the spine.

Sores occur most commonly when there are lumps or wrinkles or tears in the saddle lining *(photo 4)* or in the blanket used beneath the saddle. These

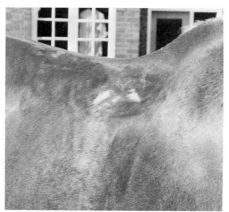

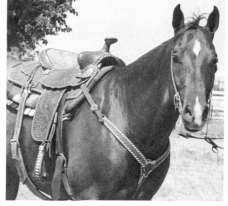

1

2

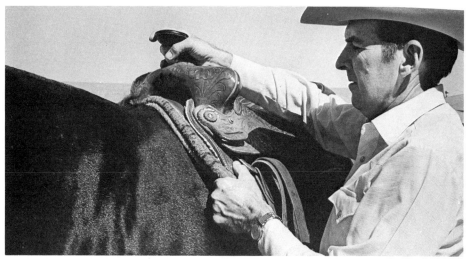

3

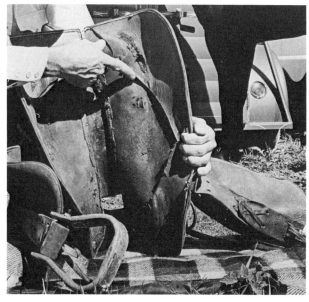

4

produce excessive pressure on a certain point, inhibiting the flow of blood to that part of the skin. Depending on the length of time the pressure is maintained, varying amounts of damage result. Two smooth pads or blankets *(photo 5)* can be used to eliminate the pressure unless the saddle is to be repaired before further use.

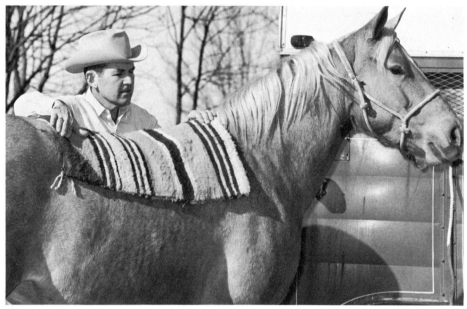

5

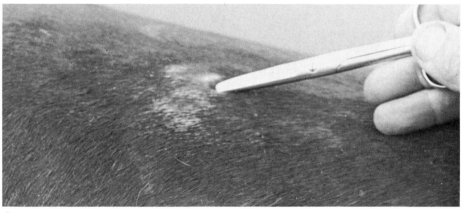

6

The damage to the horse's skin, if spotted early, may be only a slight erosion of the skin surface *(photo 6)*. If, however, pressure is allowed to continue, the size and depth of the erosion will increase, creating a nasty open sore.

Another common cause of saddle sores is dirt. The lining or blanket becomes covered with hair, dried sweat, and even mud; once again, areas of uneven pressure are set up.

Saddle sores can, of course, be caused simply by bad riding. If you sit in the saddle with more weight on one buttock than the other, or if you persistently roll around in the saddle, you can soon subject your horse to chafing and soreness. The golden rule, when mounted, is to sit square and sit still. Other causes of wounds in this area should also be inspected (insect bites, abrasions, etc.) before riding.

Girth Sores

Once again there are various causes: (1) old girths that are rough on the inside, (2) dirty girths—these chafe and produce sores, so make sure your girth is clean *(photo 7),* (3) a badly fitting saddle or a saddle set too far forward, so that the girth rubs on the skin at the back of the elbows and produces nasty sores, and (4) allergic dermatitis involving the chest and belly wall, not unusual in the warmer months.

How to Prevent Saddle and Girth Sores
After the saddle has been put on and girthed up and you are sure it is in the correct position, draw each of the horse's forelegs well forward—get in front and pull them well out *(photo 8).* This brings the skin clear into its correct position below the girth.

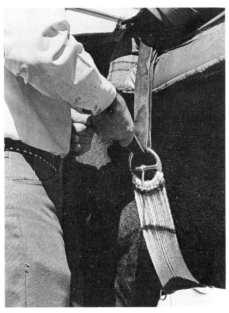

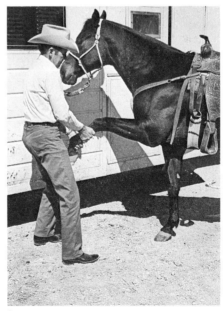

7   8

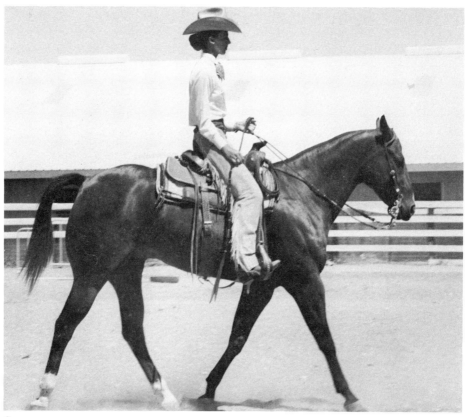

9

Even if the saddle is a perfect fit, and even if it is correctly put on, there is always some slight inhibition of the blood flow through the skin of the back. Obviously, therefore, if you are at a show or gymkhana or on a long ride, you should stop periodically—preferably every hour. Slacken the girth, raise the saddle, and allow the blood to flow freely for at least five minutes throughout the pressure area. So often one sees children at shows leaving their ponies tightly girthed while they go off for ice cream or to watch the other events. This is very bad. If you have an opportunity for a breather, give your pony's back and sides a breather also.

Make sure at all times that you have a well-fitting saddle and girth. Any experienced horseman or saddle maker can advise you.

Keep the saddle and girth particularly clean. This means that after every ride, both the saddle and girth should be sponged down and dried thoroughly, paying particular attention to the inside linings.

Sit correctly in the saddle *(photo 9)* and don't roll about.

Treatment

Treatment depends on the extent of damage, but the one thing that is always essential is rest—complete rest. A saddle sore or a girth sore will never heal if it is periodically exposed to further chafing. This is just common sense, and yet the necessity for complete rest is so often disregarded.

The rest period may extend to several weeks, or even several months, but on no account should the saddle or girth be put on until the wound is completely healed and all trace of tenderness has gone.

When the wound has healed over but is not yet haired, it is often a good idea to have the saddle "chambered" by the saddler. He will mark on the saddle lining the position of the unprotected skin. He will then take back the lining and remove some of the stuffing over the marked area. When the lining is replaced, little or no pressure will be exerted on the healed part. This is always well worth doing. A second sore on the same site will take longer to heal than the first. Often, using a foam rubber pad with the involved area "mapped" on the pad and cut out will be of some benefit.

GENERAL DISEASES
AND CONDITIONS

12. Parasites

A parasite is an organism or creature that lives on or in an animal entirely at that animal's expense. The animal on or in which the parasite lives is called the host.

There are two main types of parasites: (1) external parasites, which live on the surface of the animal and include flies, mites, mosquitoes, lice, and ticks; and (2) internal parasites, which live inside the animal and include ascarids, strongyles, bots, pinworms, tapeworms, and warbles.

External Parasites

Flies

Many species of flies trouble horses. Some are bloodsucking and cause pain; others are just a nuisance.

Stable flies, which breed in decaying vegetation around the stable, are probably the most common *(photo 1)*. They normally roost on walls, trees, and

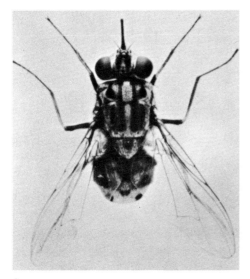

1

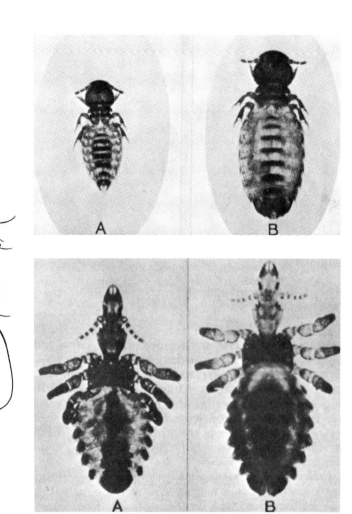

Figure 1

3

fences in the shade. Once or twice a day they come to the animal, feed vigorously for a minute or two, and return to the shade to digest their blood meal.

Houseflies and face flies, which lay eggs in fresh manure, do not bite the horse but persist around eyes, nose, and wounds.

The best prevention is sanitation and a cleanup of breeding areas. Also, the stable walls, ceiling, and fences should be sprayed periodically with one of the good residual insecticides, making sure not to get the spray on the animal or its feed.

Then the horse should be sprayed regularly (daily during the peak fly season) with one of the good animal insecticides. Since some horses dislike

70

sprays, you might have better luck wiping the material around your horse's face, using a sponge or a cloth. Be careful to keep the insecticide away from the horse's eyes. Change the insecticide you use occasionally, because flies build up a resistance to one kind.

If mosquitoes or ticks are a problem in your area, check with your veterinarian or county agent for the recommended insecticide.

Mange

This problem, caused by small mites that burrow under the skin *(figure 1),* is the most serious of the external parasites.

Mange is a contagious disease. However, although a mange-free horse may be near an infected one, it will not contract the disease unless the two rub against one another. Of course, the mites can also be picked up from box stalls, grooming tackle, fence posts, etc.

Symptoms

Mange causes intense irritation and itching. It can start anywhere but often flares up first at the tailhead or legs or at the base of the mane. The horse bites or rubs the part almost continuously; very soon, bald patches appear.

Diagnosis and Treatment

Your veterinarian should be consulted in all suspect cases. He or she can take skin scrapings, examine them under the microscope, and then supply a dressing or a bath solution to be applied daily for several days. One popular treatment is a 0.6 percent lindane and 0.5 percent toxaphene solution to be brushed into the affected area.

Mange is a reportable disease.

Lice

Lice that infest horses are of both the biting and sucking kind *(photos 2 and 3).* They are found mainly on horses that are poorly fed and neglected.

Lice are picked up in the same way as the mange mites; that is, by direct contact or from dirty box stalls, tackle, etc. Like mange, lice infestation is a contagious condition.

Symptoms

The signs of lice are identical to mange in the early stages; that is, the horse rubs, bites, and develops bare patches. However, close examination by a veteri- 71

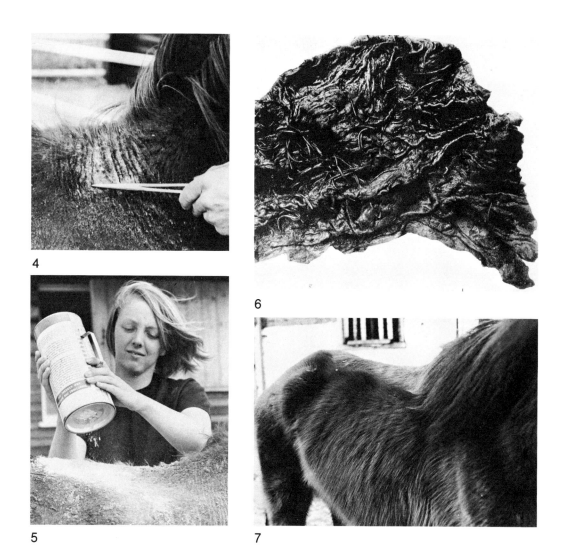

4

6

5

7

narian or by a reasonably knowledgeable horseman will show the lice and the minute white louse eggs *(photo 4)* to be found at varying distances along the hair shafts.

Treatment

There are many good baths and louse powders *(photo 5),* any one of which will kill the adult lice. However, as in mange, the dressings do not kill the eggs

72

and therefore must be repeated once a week for several weeks to kill the lice as they hatch out and before they have a chance to lay more eggs.

Prevention

Remember: A well-cared-for horse will never get lice. Good, regular feeding, exercise, and grooming will nearly always prevent the establishment of a lice infestation.

Internal Parasites

Over fifty species of internal parasites have been identified in the United States. But we will discuss here only those that are most common: ascarids, strongyles, bots, pinworms, and the less common tapeworms and warbles.

Ascarids

Ascarids, also known as roundworms, are the largest internal parasite affecting horses. The adults get as long as 8 to 12 inches and as large in diameter as a lead pencil.

Much ascarid damage is done as they progress through the horse's system. After hatching in the small intestine, the tiny worms migrate through the liver and to the lungs. Then they are coughed up, reswallowed, and again enter the small intestine to continue growing.

Mature horses develop some immunity, but foals and young horses are particularly susceptible. Foals with ascarids are often potbellied and rough-haired; they are erratic feeders and often have a persistent cough. The occasional young horse (usually eighteen months or younger) will suffer a severe impaction and/or ruptured intestine because of their presence.

Strongyles

Strongyles, which range from ¾ inch to 2 inches in length, are commonly called bloodworms, because they suck blood through the walls of the digestive tract *(photo 6)*. (Strongyles are sometimes called roundworms too.) They tend to concentrate in arteries, where they slow or stop blood flow, which in turn causes recurring colic or at least a compromised digestive system. Be aware that infected horses may have a reasonably normal appearance; not all of them noticeably lose condition as shown here *(photo 7)*. Bloodworms are easily the most common killer of horses.

73

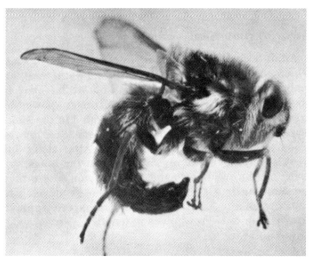

8

Bots

Botflies, which resemble small bees *(photo 8),* deposit small white eggs on the tips of hairs on the forelegs and nearby areas of the horse. These flies are very irritating to horses, causing them to stomp and sometimes run.

The eggs hatch into small larvae which the horse licks into his mouth. There the larvae burrow into the tongue or cheeks and remain for two or three weeks, apparently without causing any worry.

From the mouth, the small worms migrate to the stomach, where they develop into larger larvae and by means of their teeth attach themselves to the inside of the stomach wall *(photo 9).* After spending all winter in the stomach, they release their hold, pass out with the manure in the spring, and develop into adult flies to begin the life cycle all over again. During their stay in the stomach, they are capable of creating a gastritis (inflammation of the stomach lining) and associated digestive system problems.

Throughout the fly season, if you brush the eggs off the forelegs every day or scrape them off with a knife, the few larvae that do reach the horse's stomach will do little or no harm.

Pinworms

Pinworms, which are 2 or 3 inches when mature, spend much of their time in the rectum and come to the anal opening to lay eggs around the outside of

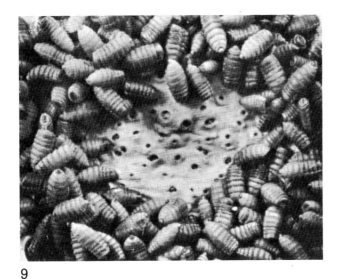

9

the anus. This results in severe irritation and itching, causing the horse to rub the tail on any stationary object. In severe infections, most of the hair on the tailhead is rubbed away.

How to Identify the Parasitized Horse

Any unthrifty horse (see *photo 7*), particularly when on pasture, should always be suspect. Bear in mind that most horses are to one degree or another parasitized. Identification of the parasite load is made by microscopic examination of fecal material.

Prevention

Adequate prevention is dependent on several factors: (1) Climatic conditions in which the horse exists (warm, humid areas favor large parasite populations). (2) The degree of exposure; that is, the density of horse population and frequency of exposure to other horses at shows, racetracks, etc.. (3) Stable and pasture management. (Continual exposure to manure maintains the life cycle of the internal parasites with the exception of bots.)

The most effective control is based on regular administration of anthelmintics. Under the best of circumstances (arid climate, few horses with lots of acres, etc.) horses should probably be dewormed twice a year. Where the population of horses is high and the concentration great, it may well be necessary to deworm every sixty days. Such a determination can be made only for the individual situation.

In any case, prevention is a function of frequent deworming and reduction of exposure (pasture rotation, when possible, and daily stall cleaning). With each year, new drugs are being introduced; therefore, it is now possible to use a variety of safe anthelmintics so as to avoid drug resistance within a population of parasites.

Treatment

In badly affected cases, treatment is very much a job for your veterinarian. After identifying the involved parasite and estimating the extent of infestation, he or she will then prescribe the appropriate anthelmintic. You may also choose to supplement the diet of the involved animal, in addition to the deworming, if the horse's condition warrants it.

Tapeworms

The tapeworm is a commensal parasite, meaning that it develops in the horse's intestines but causes no known damage to them. It merely lives in the intestinal tract and represents at best a questionable situation.

The tapeworm lays eggs in its own tail, then detaches the egg-laden tail, which is passed out onto the pastures.

The eggs hatch out into minute larvae which are eaten by small nonparasitic mites. Inside the mites the larvae develop into cysts.

The horse eats the mites with the grass. In the horse's intestines, the cysts rupture and develop very quickly into adult tapeworms—male and female— which copulate and start the cycle once more.

Warbles

The warble or grub is not nearly so common in the horse as in cattle, but when it does get onto the horse, it can cause considerable pain and damage.

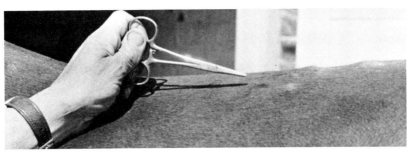

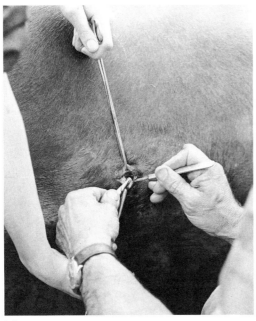

11

Like the botfly, the warble fly likes warm weather and appears in the summertime. The eggs are laid at the *base* of the hairs and on the lower parts of all *four* legs. There the eggs hatch out into minute larvae which penetrate the skin and migrate throughout the body until they eventually arrive at the back, frequently just under the saddle area.

They appear as small painful lumps under the skin of the back *(photo 10)*. In cattle the mature larvae pass out through the skin to develop into a new generation of flies, but in horses the larvae often die under the skin, producing either an abscess or a fistula. When this happens, they have to be removed by surgical means *(photo 11)*.

Even after surgery, a painful sore remains which may take considerable time to heal sufficiently for the horse to be put back to work.

Prevention and Treatment

Preventing warble infestation in horses is almost impossible unless the horse is at stable on a farm where cattle are strictly treated against the fly.

As for treatment, it must be left to your veterinarian to decide whether surgical removal is necessary. In the majority of cases they are best left completely alone, provided that the horse can be adequately rested.

77

13. Ringworm

As in man and in other animals, ringworm in the horse *(photo 1)* is a contagious disease. It is caused by several different fungal organisms.

The disease is the result of direct contact with an infected or "carrier" horse. A carrier is an animal that conveys the fungus without showing any clinical signs of the disease. Recovered animals sometimes remain carriers. The horse may also pick up the fungus from an infected box stall or a trailer or from infected grooming kits, horse blankets, saddles, etc.

Symptoms

First of all, the hair will appear to stand up and rise in small circular patches.

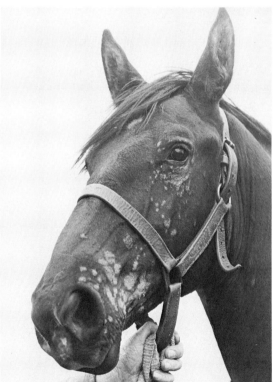

1

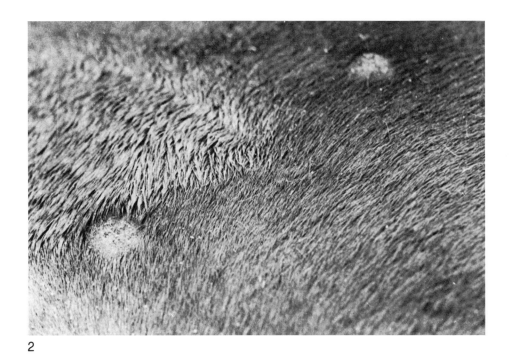

2

Then the hair in the patches will fall out and leave circular bald areas *(photo 2)*. The circular spots may eventually become crusty or septic.

The fungi that cause ringworm are aerobes; that is, they require oxygen, so that when the lesions become crusted over, the ones in the center die and the live fungi keep working outward away from the center, thereby producing the typical ringworm appearance. The fungi are therefore to be found in greatest concentration at the outside or periphery of the circular areas.

Diagnosis is made on the symptoms, but it can be confirmed definitely only by the examination of skin scrapings in a laboratory.

Treatment

An infected or suspect pony or horse should be isolated.

All grooming equipment, blankets, feeding utensils, etc., must be regularly disinfected with an iodine preparation or comparable antiseptic and kept for that specific animal only.

The lesions should be dressed once a week for three weeks, using a reliable nonirritant antifungal application *(photo 3)* which will be supplied by your veterinarian. It is a good idea first to scrub the lesions with hot water and soda to remove the crusts and expose the fungi to the effects of the dressing.

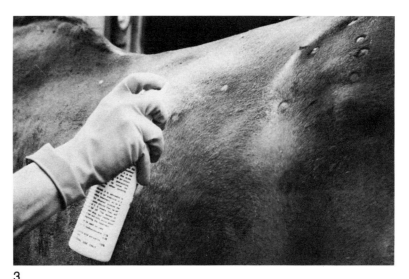

3

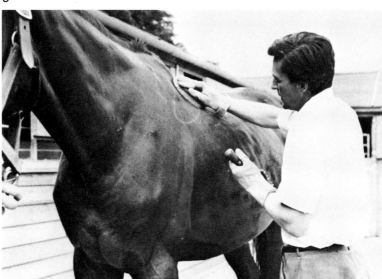

4

One important point to remember: Horse ringworm is infectious to man, so be very careful with your hands and nails. Always wear rubber gloves when grooming the infected animal *(photo 4)* and keep the gloves soaking in the disinfectant with the grooming tackle.

A feed supplement that contains an antifungal drug, called griesofulvin, is now available and is very effective.

14. Tail Rubbing, or Itchy Tail

This is a comparatively common condition in ponies and horses of all ages, particularly during the summer. It can be caused by mange mites, pinworms, fungi, or allergies.

The most common cause in this country is an allergic phenomenon resulting from biting insects.

Symptoms

These are unmistakable—the horse starts rubbing the base of his tail against gateways or fence posts. The affected areas become devoid of hair *(photo 1),* and if rubbing is continued, the skin may become inflamed and raw.

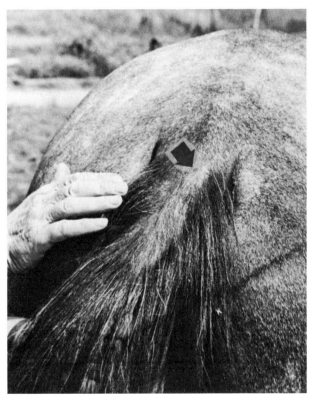

1

Treatment

Get your veterinarian on the job at once, to check the feces for pinworm eggs and examine the area for mange mites. The mange mite, however, is difficult to diagnose, and it usually takes several days to determine if a fungus is present. For this reason, the veterinarian may use a "shotgun" treatment: recommend worming the horse, if this hasn't been done recently, and treat with a fungicide, an insecticide, and another fungicide, all over a period of six to eight days. These solutions are applied as a bath around the tailhead and on the tail itself. They should drench the area well enough to penetrate the hair and saturate the skin. In the event of an allergic phenomenon, an effort will have to be made to cut down on exposure to biting insects by judicious use of insecticides, stabling management, etc. Often the animal will have to be put on antiallergic medication, such as cortisone, during the high insect-biting months.

15. Tetanus

Tetanus, often called lockjaw, is one of the greatest potential enemies of the horse, pony, mule, and donkey.

It is caused by the *Clostridium tetani,* a bacterium called a sporulating germ because it surrounds itself with a thick protective coat to form what the scientist describes as a "spore." *Figure 1* shows sporulating tetanus bacilli in a stained microscopic slide of pus.

The tetanus spore can lie dormant in the ground for many years, provided it has available a minimal amount of moisture. For this reason, the germ is more often found on moist, arable, or heavy land than on old, light, dry, permanent pasture.

Figure 1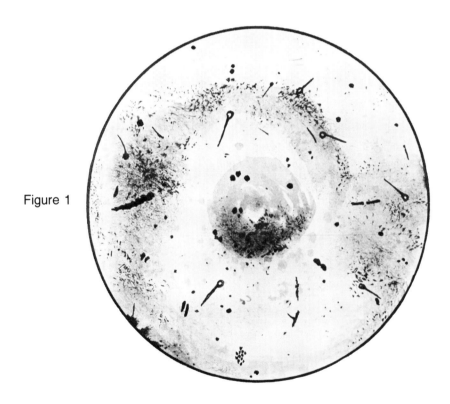

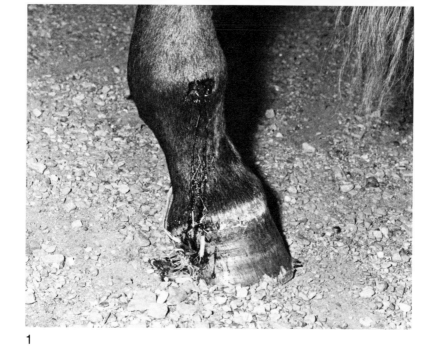

1

Method of Infection

A deep puncture wound provides the ideal spot for the tetanus spores to get to work *(photo 1)*. In such a wound there is little or no air and the spores, being what we call anaerobes (bacteria that live in the absence of oxygen), will throw off their protective coats and start to multiply on the spot. The germs do not enter the bloodstream, but they excrete a poisonous waste product called a toxin. This toxin travels from the nerve endings along the nerves toward the spinal cord, playing havoc with the nerves' true functions. The resulting symptoms vary according to the amount of toxin and the extent of the nerve involvement.

Symptoms

The first sign usually seen in horses is that the head is held forward and the nostrils are slightly distended, giving the muzzle a square appearance *(figure 2)*.

Figure 2

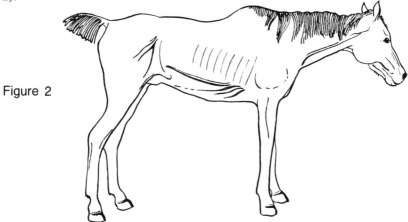

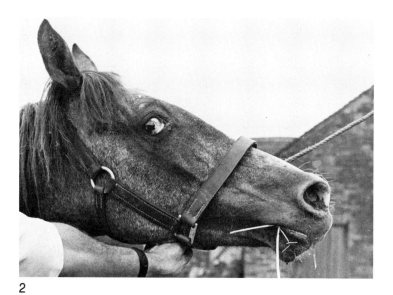

2

The legs are often placed slightly wider than normal, particularly the hind legs, with the hocks turned outward and the tail raised. When made to move, the animal walks stiffly as though afraid.

If the horse is startled, the third eyelid will often flash across the eye *(photo 2)*. (The third eyelid is referred to as the membrana nictitans.) This is highly suggestive that the animal is suffering from tetanus.

As the symptoms advance, the horse may become wildly excited. He may have great difficulty in breathing, and the jaws may become clamped, with the facial muscles rigid and hard. Needless to say, when this happens, the patient is unable to eat or drink.

Treatment

Treatment is rarely successful, especially if the symptoms are at all advanced. In most cases euthanasia is indicated, but the veterinarian is the correct person to confirm the diagnosis and make the final decision.

Prevention

This is one disease which should always be immunized against. Fortunately, a highly efficient injection against tetanus is available.

The best method of control is to have the animals injected with two doses of tetanus toxoid at monthly intervals, and a booster dose every year thereafter. This is the ideal routine and should be followed religiously by every horse or pony owner.

In addition, whenever there is a puncture wound, a tetanus booster should also be given by the veterinarian. This gives immediate protection and doubles the insurance.

85

16. Encephalomyelitis

There are three strains of *equine encephalomyelitis,* sometimes called "blind staggers" or "sleeping sickness," in the United States—Eastern, Western, and Venezuelan (VEE). In general, the epidemics of the Eastern strain have occurred in the East and the Gulf Coast states, the Western strain in the West and Midwest and the Venezuelan strain in the Southwest, mainly Texas. However, because so many horses now are transported from state to state, you can't count on any one strain's being limited to its original epidemic area. Some states are known to have two or three strains.

All three strains are viruses; they are slightly different, but only laboratory tests can definitely distinguish the difference. The viruses are harbored in birds and are carried to horses by mosquitoes or other bloodsucking insects. The horse is considered a "dead-end host," as the disease is not transferable to another animal except possibly in the case of VEE. Contaminated hypodermic needles can spread it. People sometimes contract it from mosquitoes.

Symptoms

The first signs are marked depression and a high fever. Later, you may notice the lower lip drooping, the eyeballs oscillating, a reluctance of the animal to move, and poor coordination *(photo 1).* Often, the horse staggers (thus the name "blind staggers"), and some horses have even walked through barn walls. Horses in the advanced stages of VEE often walk in a circle with their heads lowered *(photo 2).* Once the patient gets down, it sometimes digs a trench in the ground by pawing with its front feet.

Treatment

Very few animals with the Eastern and Venezuelan strains survive, and the few that do often have permanent brain damage. Usually, by the time you notice clinical signs of the disease, it's too late to use an immunization serum. So about all you or the veterinarian can do is keep the animal comfortable, protect it from injury, and try to maintain a balance of body fluids and electrolytes.

Western equine encephalomyelitis is not quite as deadly—only about half the victims die, compared to about 90 percent mortality from the other two

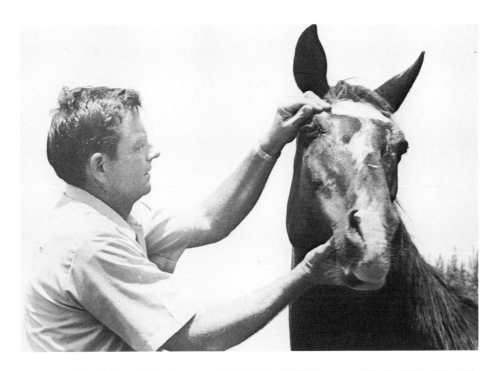

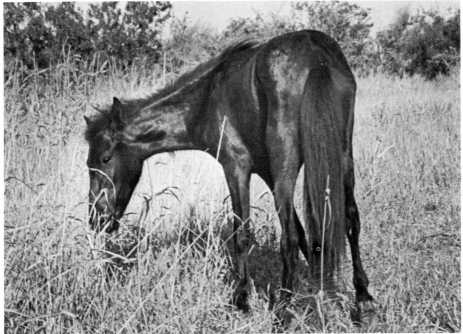

2

strains. There is no specific drug for this but, if caught in the early stages, treatment with an immunization serum may help. In addition, your veterinarian will try to maintain the proper fluid and electrolyte balance and to lower the patient's temperature. You should keep the horse as comfortable as possible, protect it from injury, and try to keep it standing.

Prevention

Fortunately, we have vaccines that are quite effective in immunizing horses against all three strains of equine encephalomyelitis. These should be given in the spring or early summer, before the mosquito season.

Since the Eastern and Western strains have been recognized for at least seventy-five years, bivalent vaccines have been developed, which means that they protect against both strains. Two injections are required, seven to fourteen days apart, every year.

Since the first epidemic of Venezuelan equine encephalomyelitis (VEE) in the United States was in 1971, this vaccine is much newer and the duration of its effectiveness is not fully known. A single injection, recommended for all horses over six months of age, will immunize for at least two years and can be given at the same time as the bivalent vaccine for the other two strains. Foals in high-risk areas should be vaccinated when three months old and revaccinated after weaning.

Another preventive measure, particularly important in high-risk areas, is to control the mosquitoes and other bloodsucking insects that carry the disease.

17. Urticaria, or Hives

Urticaria is an allergic condition, occasionally known as "nettle rash." It is very difficult to describe exactly what is meant by the term "allergy," but, generally speaking, an allergy occurs when some external factor disagrees with some normal factor within the animal. For example, stings from certain plants (such as nettles, *photo 1*) or from flies and insects may bring it on, or changes in feeding, particularly when the protein is increased.

Urticaria is not generally serious, but it can be very alarming. Usually in veterinary practice it comes through as a panic call, and almost invariably by the time we get there the symptoms have subsided.

Symptoms

There will be raised blotches or weals over the entire body *(photo 2),* usually most marked around the head and neck and under the belly and tail. Occasionally the head and throat regions swell to twice the normal size, and the horse may have difficulty in breathing freely. The temperature and pulse remain normal.

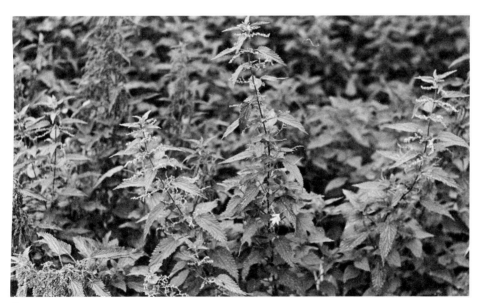

1

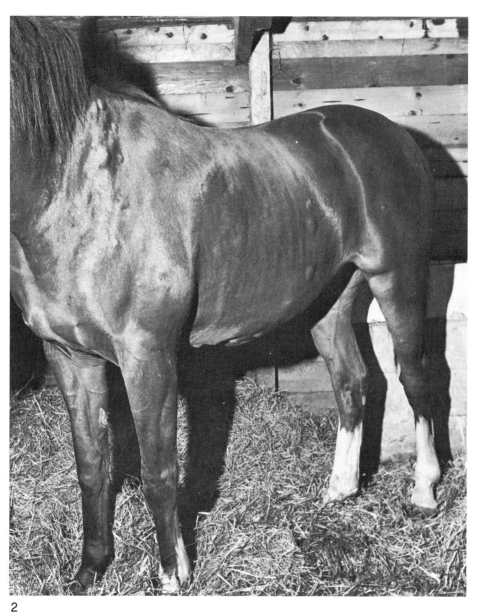

2

Treatment

      Left alone, the weals will generally reduce in size, assuming that the cause has been removed. The condition usually responds quickly to appropriate medications, such as antihistamine, cortisone, or other similar drugs.

18. Purpura Hemorrhagica

The specific cause of purpura is unknown at this time, though it is considered an allergic phenomenon. It generally follows a respiratory infection and is thought to be an allergic reaction to the presence of whatever organism initiated the original infection. The two respiratory diseases that are occasionally followed by purpura hemorrhagica are equine flu and strangles.

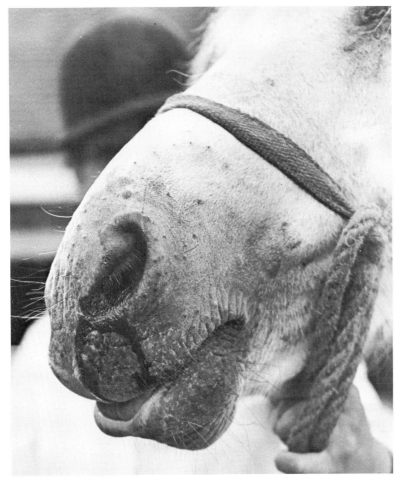

1

Symptoms

The first noticeable sign is generally the appearance of a swelling between the front legs, or along the floor of the belly, or on any—or all—of the four legs, usually at the top. Occasionally the head is affected and the nose swells up. The purpura swellings, or lumps, are characteristic in that they generally have well-defined edges. They are not painful and will pit on pressure.

Inside the nostrils, petechiae (minute red hemorrhages) appear. Similar petechiae occur throughout the entire body, and there may be a bloody or pink-colored discharge from the nostrils *(photo 1)* and from the other natural openings.

The temperature rises several degrees but may drop back to normal or subnormal after a few days. The pulse is accelerated.

The horse is usually extremely sick and may refuse to eat or drink.

Treatment

There is no known specific cure, and the condition is often fatal. However, there are many lines of treatment and some animals do recover, so your veterinarian should be consulted immediately. If the horse keeps eating, its chances of recovery are enhanced, though convalescence is invariably prolonged.

It has been my experience that complete recovery from purpura hemorrhagica takes a comparatively long time.

19. Melanoma

A melanoma is a small growth (tumor) which is frequently found in gray or white horses. This tumor type may or may not be malignant; that is, it may reach a certain size and character and remain as such, or it may become highly invasive and involve multiple tissues. Its behavior is not very predictable. All such swellings and tumors should be examined by your veterinarian.

Symptoms

Usually, multiple small hard lumps develop around the anus and tail base *(photo 1)*. Most will generally cause little or no discomfort unless they ulcerate. However, they may continue to spread internally.

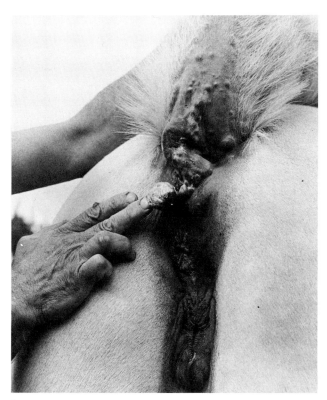

1

These tumors also frequently affect the parotid gland (below the ear behind the jaw) and may at times be found in the region of the sheath, the udder, and occasionally on the legs.

Persistent hind-leg lameness in a gray or a white horse should always alert the owner to the possibility of an internal malignant melanoma.

Generally speaking, since malignant melanomas have been reported involving many different tissues throughout the body, the symptoms will vary with the location and the type of tissue involved.

Treatment

There is none. Your veterinarian will be required to diagnose the internal melanoma and will advise accordingly. When the growths are external and are causing no discomfort or lameness, they should be left alone. If they become malignant, most horses are humanely destroyed, since present-day cancer therapy is not practical or effective for horses at this time.

20. Warts (Papillomas)

As in all animals, warts on horses and ponies are a nuisance, to say the least, especially during the summer when the flies seek them out for special attention. The persistent irritation of the fly bites makes the animal restless and bad tempered.

It is now fairly well established that warts are caused by viruses. The viruses have not yet been identified, but vaccines can be prepared against them.

Treatment

Even the smallest wart or group of warts should be treated without delay *(photo 1).* Modern wart dressings are extremely effective, provided the mass is not overwhelming. The appropriate dressing will be supplied by your veterinarian.

If the infection becomes widespread, the veterinarian can send off a sample of the wart tissue and have what is called an autogenous vaccine prepared against the virus.

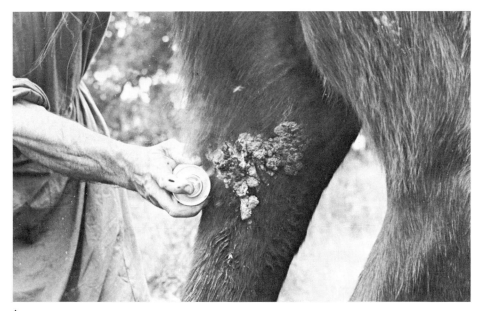

1

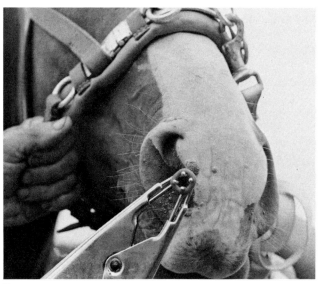
2

When the wart is persistent or in a vital area of the horse's anatomy such as the genitals, the veterinarian may have to remove it surgically.

Papillomas and warts can be ligated—that is, tied off so that the blood supply is stopped—and perhaps the best form of ligature is the rubber ring used with and applied by the elastrator *(photo 2)*. However, when this method is used, the horse must always be injected against tetanus, since the wound caused by the elastrator rubber ring provides an ideal focus for the growth of tetanus bacteria.

HEAD REGION

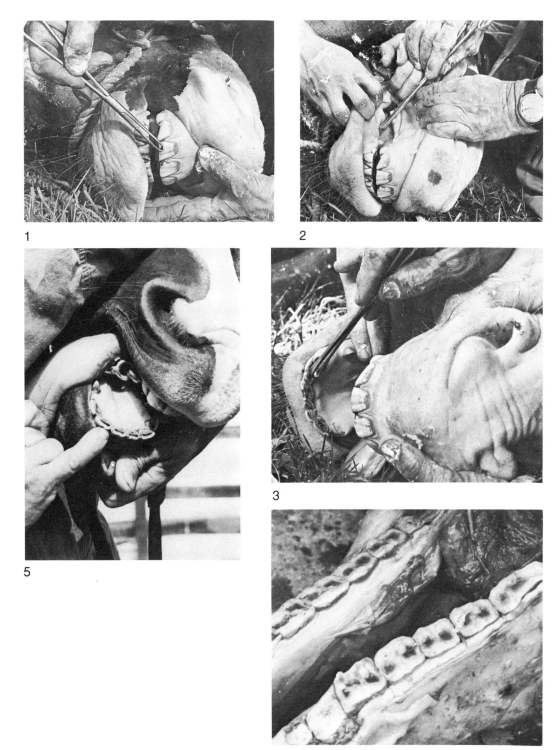

1

2

3

4

5

21. The Teeth

An intelligent assessment of a horse's age can be made only by having a sound general knowledge of the teeth.

Broadly speaking, there are two types of teeth—those at the front called the incisors *(photo 1)* and those at the rear called the molars.

The portions of bare gums between the incisors and the molars are called the "bars," and it is on these areas that the bit should rest *(photo 2)*.

Horses' teeth differ from those of humans in that the horse does not chew his food but grinds it; therefore, the surfaces of the teeth are flat to allow the grinding *(photo 3)*.

When a horse has all his teeth (we call it a "full mouth"), there are six incisors on the top jaw and six incisors on the lower jaw. We describe these as two centrals, two laterals, and two corners.

There are six molars on each side, top and bottom *(photo 4)*.

How to Tell a Horse's Age

When born, a foal has its two central incisors through the gum or just on the point of coming through.

The two lateral incisors appear at about five weeks, and the corners at approximately eight months, so by eight months the foal has a complete set of front or incisor teeth.

The front three molars on both sides are there at birth or within two weeks.

All these teeth are temporary or milk teeth and are replaced, as time goes on, by the permanent teeth. The replacing is consistent, and it is by the replacement of the incisor teeth that the horse's age can be accurately assessed.

The two central permanents come up through the gums at 2½ years and are in wear at 3 years.

The two laterals are up at 3½ years and are in wear at 4 years.

The corners are up at 4½ years and in wear at 5 years. At this age the horse is said to be "rough-mouthed."

All these incisor teeth have black concentric rings or cavities on their tables *(photo 5),* and it is from these that age is determined during the next three years.

99

The cavities in the central incisors disappear at 6 years; those in the laterals at 7 years and those in the corners at 8 years. At this age and thereafter a horse is said to be aged, or "smooth-mouthed."

Estimation of age from 8 years onward requires considerable skill and professional experience.

At 8 to 10 years a dark line appears at the top of the outside of the upper corner incisor (photo 6). This line (the so-called "galvaynes groove") extends downward with each year and reaches the bottom of the tooth at about 20 years.

From 10 years onward the incisors also start to protrude forward, and the tables of the teeth, instead of being almost circular, become oval—then triangular—from front to back (photo 7). It is from the shape of the tables of the incisors that an experienced veterinarian can tell at once whether a horse is old or young. It is well, therefore, for the reader to examine the photographs carefully so that he or she will be less likely to be duped. Study photo 7, then refer back to the ovoid shape of the incisor tables in the young horse (photo 5). Every knowledgeable horse owner should be able to tell at a glance whether he or she is dealing with a young or an old horse.

Care of the Teeth

The horse, remember, grinds his food and thereby wears down the molar teeth. The teeth continue to grow from the gums to compensate for the wear, so that they always remain, or should remain, at the same level.

The tables of the lower molars slope downward and outward, and the tables of the upper molars slope inward and upward to match them.

The result of the continual grinding is that the inside edges of the lower molars may become very sharp (photo 8) and may scratch or cut the tongue; the outside edges of the upper molars also become sharp and can scratch or cut the cheek. In either case, the horse does not eat properly and often "quids"; that is, he drops portions of partly ground food onto the floor or ground.

Unlike the teeth of humans, horses' teeth are rarely subject to decay, but their teeth should be checked for other conditions and irregularities. The molars should be examined at least once a year by a veterinarian, who will rasp smooth any sharp edges or points. With the help of a device to hold the mouth ajar (photo 9), this is a simple and painless operation, and the majority of horses will stand quietly while it is being done.

Sometimes, in older horses particularly, a molar may grow excessively long, usually because of a broken or shed tooth on the opposite arcade of teeth. When this happens, the offending molar will have to be dealt with frequently. It is either filed or, in some cases, sheared.

100

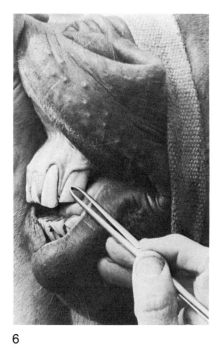

6

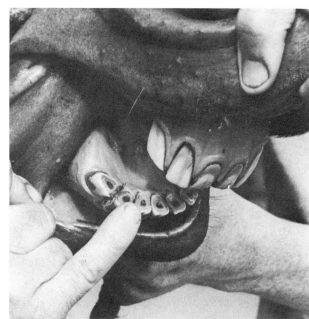

7

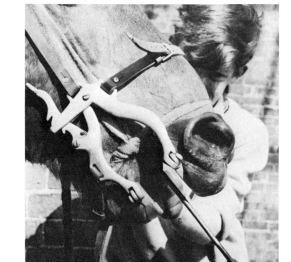

9

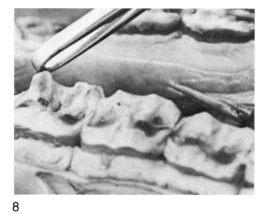

8

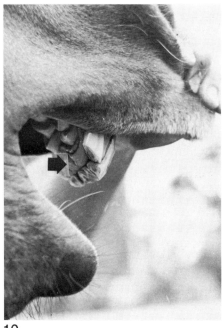

10

Lampas

Lampas is a swelling of the horse's hard palate—the roof of his mouth. While it is not a condition directly affecting the teeth, it is sometimes first discovered only when the teeth are given veterinary attention.

It occurs most commonly in young horses when they are first introduced to hard feed (grain) and have not yet learned how to manage it properly in their mouths. The irritation and resultant edema of the palate can be quite severe *(photo 10),* causing the horse to go off his feed and even to lose condition, simply because it hurts his mouth to eat.

At one time lampas was treated by lancing the swollen palate and rubbing salt into the knife wound. Luckily, the remedy today is less drastic: Reduce the ration at first and soften the grain by soaking.

22. The Eye

Eye injuries should always be regarded as serious until proven otherwise. You are well advised to have any suspect eye problems examined by your veterinarian.

Simple Anatomy of the Eye

The eye comprises a number of distinct parts (see *figure 1,* a vertical cross section). At the front surface is the *cornea,* which is a clear membrane, almost like a window with a microfine pane.

Behind the cornea is the *iris.* The iris dilates or contracts according to the intensity of the light it is exposed to.

Between the iris and the cornea is a space containing fluid. This is called the *anterior chamber.*

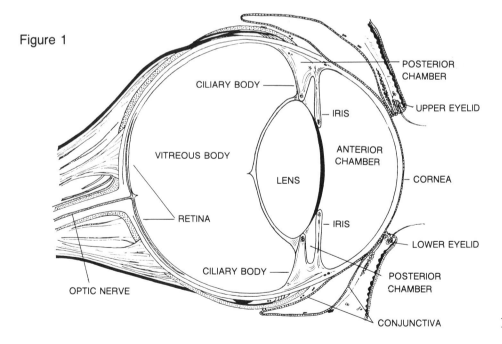

Figure 1

103

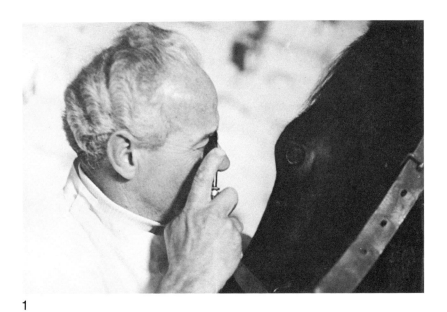

1

The space between the iris and the *lens* is called the *posterior chamber.* The fluid within the anterior and posterior chambers communicates freely through the pupil, the central opening in the iris.

The lens, by way of a specialized muscle mechanism, can relax and become thicker, or tense and become thinner, in this way allowing the eye to focus on near or distant objects.

Behind the lens, the cavity of the eyeball is filled with a very clear semisolid substance called the *vitreous body* (or *uvea*).

The cavity of the eyeball, behind the lens, is lined by the *retina,* where everything the horse sees is recorded and transmitted to the brain.

Unlike humans, the horse has a third eyelid originating from the inside corner—the nictitating membrane.

How to Examine the Eye

To do this properly, it is essential to have the horse in a completely dark stall or to wait until nighttime. It is no use just turning the horse with his back end to the windows; the stall must be dark.

A veterinarian with an ophthalmoscope *(photo 1)* can examine the eye completely, but the layman can make a very satisfactory examination without this instrument. The routine is as follows:

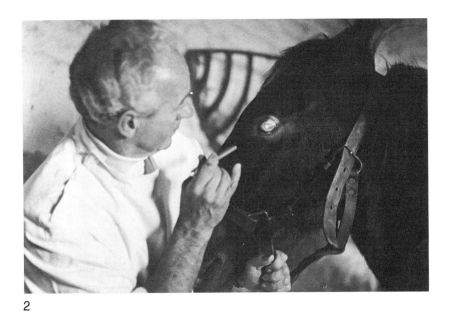

2

Take a small pencil flashlight. Shine it into the eye directly in front and then sideways *(photo 2)*. In this way you can make sure that the whole surface of the cornea is absolutely clear.

Next, shine the light straight at the eye and watch for the pupil to contract. Move the light gradually away: the pupil should expand. This indicates that the animal is seeing and is reacting normally to light.

Using the small penlight, hold it in front of the eye. You should be able to discern three images of the light: one on the surface of the cornea, one on the front surface of the lens, and one at the back of the lens. If there is opacity of the lens (cataract formation), you will probably be able to discern only two images. In the event that you are able to see only one image, it probably indicates that there is some reason for opacity in the anterior chamber of the eye, obscuring the lens.

Corneal Opacity

Opacity, or clouding of the surface of the eye, is one of the more common equine eye conditions *(photo 3)*.

It is usually caused by an injury, perhaps the result of being flicked by the branches of a tree or injured by a whip. There may be a puncture or a scratch on the corneal surface.

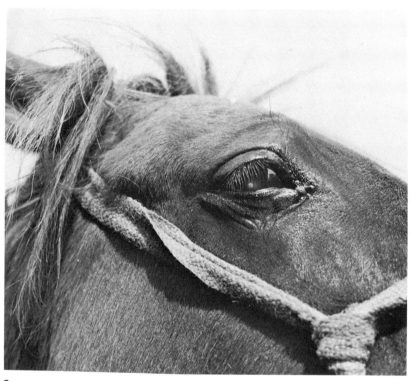

3

Treatment

Send for your veterinarian immediately. Modern antibiotic eye dressings are extremely efficient, and any delay in application can mean the loss of an eye, especially if the cornea is punctured.

Prognosis

In the vast majority of cases the sight will not be lost, but often a scar— a bluish-white mark shaped like a round dot or a minute whiplash—will remain permanently on the corneal surface. This may constitute an unsoundness, depending on the size and degree of opacity.

Cataract

In cataract formation, a clouding of the lens occurs; it becomes gray and opaque. (One can liken it to looking through a frosted windowpane.) Using a penlight as described under How to Examine the Eye, you will not be able to find the third image. Fortunately, cataract formation is reasonably uncommon in a horse, though it can occasionally be congenital and can affect one or both eyes.

Treatment

Surgical correction is not useful at this time, which means basically that there is no treatment.

Tumor of the Third Eyelid

On the membrana nictitans—the nictitating or third eyelid—a small tumor occasionally grows *(photo 4)*. It is often an invasive tumor (that is, invading associated tissues of the eye), but it is seldom malignant.

Treatment

The growth must be removed by a veterinarian. If there is little or no local invasion, surgical removal is relatively simple and usually successful. (Be aware, however, that some tumors do tend to recur.)

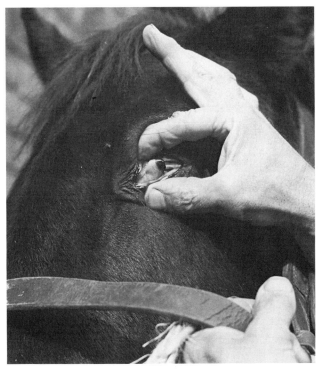

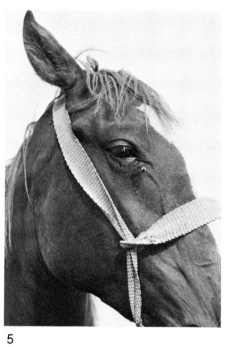

5

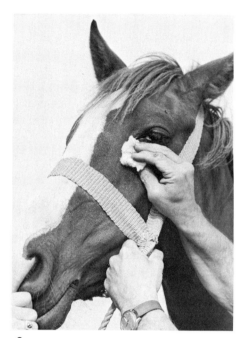

6

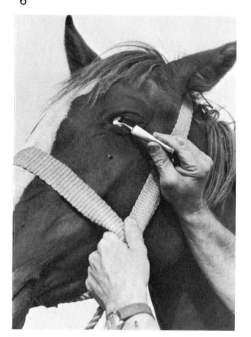

7

Conjunctivitis

Conjunctivitis, or inflammation of the conjunctiva, is by far the most common condition of the horse's eye *(photo 5)*. It frequently happens when the horse is on pasture, particularly in warm weather. Pollen dust or other irritants get into the eye and produce an inflammation. Flies are attracted, which further irritate the eye.

Symptoms

Tears run from the eye, the lids may swell, and the exposed mucous membranes become reddish. When infection starts, the eye discharge becomes pussy or purulent, giving rise to the condition we call purulent conjunctivitis. The pus dries, and if the condition is not treated promptly, crusts and sores form which attract increasing numbers of flies.

Treatment

Get your veterinarian to diagnose the condition and prescribe treatment immediately.

Prevention

This is one common condition that can be prevented by good management.

Examine the horse's eyes regularly. If the eyes are dirty, clean them with a piece of cotton soaked in warm saline solution *(photo 6)*. Dry them thoroughly and smear the lids and around the eyes with an antibiotic oil or ointment, either of which can be obtained from your veterinarian. Care must be taken to avoid damaging the eye, so always be careful when applying any medication there.

If the eyes are clear, there is no need to use the saline solution; merely spread the antibiotic around the lids and especially in the internal corners. *(photo 7)*.

109

23. Sinuses and Sinusitis

Sinuses (bony cavities) are found in the head region of horses as well as in human beings. On each side of the horse's head there are three sinuses or air spaces (*figure 1,* showing a lateral view of the skull with the sinuses opened). They are bounded on the outside by the bones that form the skull, and on the inside they are separated by the nasal septum—a cartilaginous ridge running down the center of the head from the brain.

The sinuses are lined with mucous membrane.

The top sinus is the *frontal sinus.* In the floor of this sinus there is an opening which communicates with the sinus below it—the *superior maxillary sinus.*

The superior maxillary sinus lies just below the eye on either side, and each communicates with the nasal cavity.

Below this and running along the cheek is the *inferior maxillary sinus.* This sinus is largely filled by the roots of the teeth which jut up into it. As the horse or pony grows older and the teeth wear down and protrude farther into the mouth, the inferior maxillary sinus becomes more of an air space.

The inferior maxillary sinus also communicates with the nasal cavity.

Figure 1

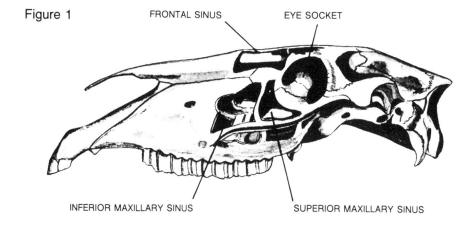

FRONTAL SINUS   EYE SOCKET

INFERIOR MAXILLARY SINUS   SUPERIOR MAXILLARY SINUS

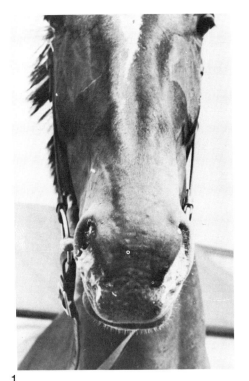

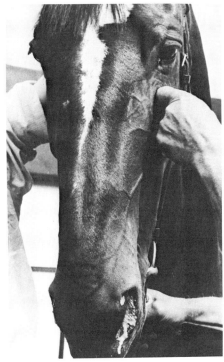

1

2

Sinus Infection

Following a severe attack of strangles or other respiratory illness, the horse may occasionally have an infection involving these sinuses. But the most prominent cause of sinus infection is diseased teeth which communicate with the sinus. The infection is indicated by pus that continually drops from one nostril or occasionally from both *(photo 1)*. The pus may stream out when the horse's head is held low or when he is grazing. Generally the material which is being passed through the nostrils is extremely malodorous.

Tapping with one knuckle on the bone just below the eye will often cause the horse to evince pain *(photo 2)*.

Treatment

Usually such cases are put on high levels of an appropriate antibiotic; in the event that the problem continues or does not respond to the antibiotic, 111

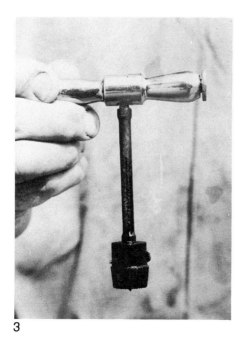

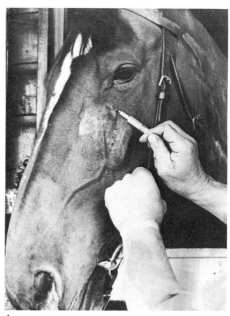

3

4

surgical intervention is required. Surgical treatment consists of trephining (making a circular hole) directly over the sinus. The trephine is a special surgical instrument used only for this purpose *(photo 3).*

The trephining can be carried out under a local anesthetic *(photo 4),* with the horse standing. It is generally done just below the eye into the superior maxillary sinus *(photo 5).*

It is usually not necessary to open into the frontal sinus, even though it may be affected, because any pus in the frontal sinus will drain through into the superior maxillary sinus.

The sinuses are then flushed out daily through the trephine hole, using a stirrup pump and a bucket of boiled water containing the correct concentration of a nonirritant antiseptic or of an antibiotic *(photo 6).* The veterinarian will do this the first time and give you instructions on continuing with it.

The antiseptic or antibiotic solution swills around the frontal and superior maxillary sinus, passes through into the nasal cavity and passages, and is discharged at the nostrils.

Should the infection be in the inferior maxillary sinus (possibly caused by an infected or split tooth), it can be treated either by trephining into the sinus or by breaking down the very thin wall, or septum, between it and the superior maxillary sinus and once again washing through from the original hole.

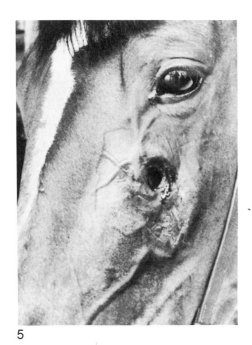 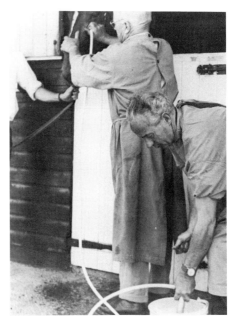

5

It is absolutely essential to keep the trephined hole very firmly plugged with sterile cotton or gauze *(photo 7);* otherwise, it will heal so rapidly that, within a few days, you will be unable to get the nozzle of your syringe or pump into it.

During the period of daily flushing, it is an advantage to give the horse a course of antibiotic injections intramuscularly.

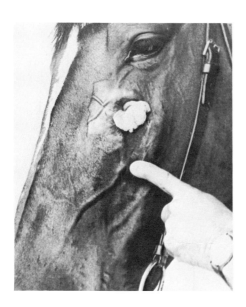

24. Facial Paralysis

This condition is caused by an injury to the facial nerve (the VII cranial). This nerve comes directly from the brain and emerges from the skull near the base of the ear. Its branches control muscles of facial expression and movements of the ear.

Although usually caused by an injury under the horse's ear or along the side of the face, facial paralysis occasionally arises secondary to a strangles abscess of the parotid lymph node, which lies just below the ear.

Symptoms

The lower lip usually droops at one side *(photo 1)*. The horse may slobber when drinking. The lips are commonly drawn toward the sound side.

The eye on the side opposite to the drooping lip may appear markedly smaller than the other.

Treatment

Such injuries are difficult to treat, depending on the cause. More often than not, the problem is temporary, unless the nerve has been severed; however, it may take up to two years for the horse to return to normal appearance. Occasionally, the defect remains permanent but, though unsightly, it rarely if ever impairs the animal's usefulness.

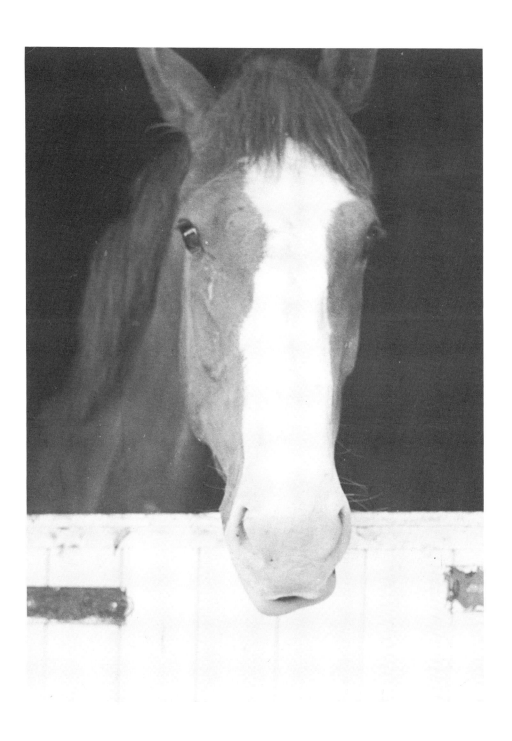

25. Itchy Ears

Sometimes a horse or a pony will show considerable irritation and distress by rubbing his ears against trees or posts and stamping his feet angrily, almost as though he has colic *(photo 1)*. Such horses can be very disagreeable and often difficult to bridle and handle in the area of the head.

Closer examination of the ears may reveal a black waxy discharge. A horse or a pony strongly resents his ears' being touched. In the summer, flies, attracted by the smell of the discharge, will be massed around the areas and will give the horse no rest.

The cause or causes are not always easily established, but in most cases the condition probably results from insect bites. Swabs can be taken from the ear contents and examined microscopically *(photo 2)*.

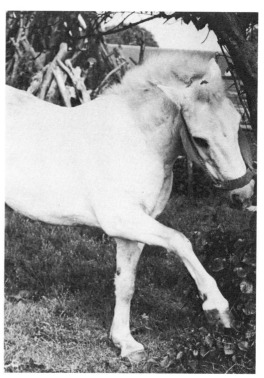

1

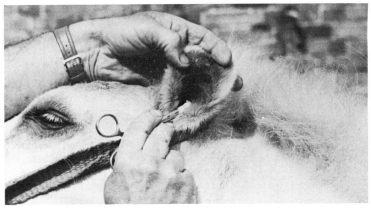

2

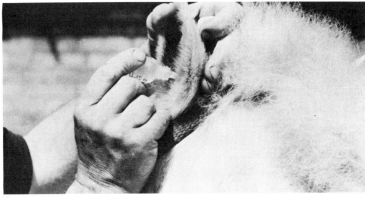

3

Treatment

Again, this is a job for your veterinarian. Assuming that a foreign body and/or infection has been ruled out, he or she will probably dress the ears with a benzyl benzoate dressing, certainly one containing an active ingredient against mites *(photo 3)*. The ears will require three dressings at intervals of five to seven days.

Keep the animal stabled or in a small lot, where it is possible to control the fly infestation. This commonsense precaution will help considerably in clearing up the condition quickly.

Prevention

The best prevention is prompt veterinary treatment at first sight of irritation. Remember, itchy ears can be kept under control, and the sooner treatment is started, the better it is for both the horse and the veterinarian.

117

26. Poll Evil and Fistulous Withers

Poll evil and fistulous withers occur when the bursa at the top of the poll, or the one at the height of the withers, becomes inflamed.

It is usually caused by an injury (often the result of mistreatment), which may be complicated by an infection.

Symptoms

There is a well-marked swelling. In the case of fistulous withers the swelling is usually in front of the upper part of the shoulder *(photo 1);* in poll evil, of course, the swelling is at the poll.

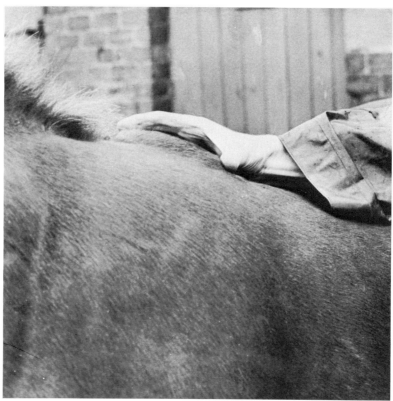

1

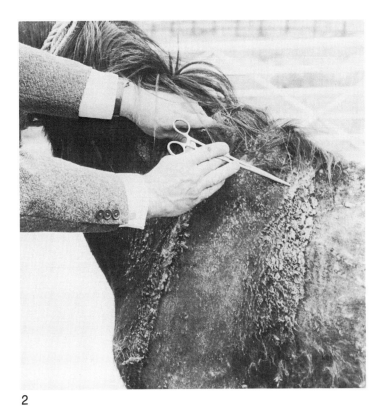

2

If the bursa is infected, it will eventually open to the outside, *(photo 2),* discharging a foul-smelling exudate. The discharge from poll evil streaks down the forehead beside the foretop.

Treatment

When poll evil is discovered, the horse should be relieved of halter and bridle. For fistulous withers the same applies to saddle and collar. Rest may be the only treatment needed.

If the condition worsens, a veterinarian should be consulted to determine the most appropriate treatment, which may range from medication to surgery. His or her concern will be to shorten the long healing process, as tissue damage may be quite extensive, and also involves the dorsal spinous processes of the underlying vertebrae.

Warning: If the swelling breaks, avoid contact with the discharge. The Brucella organism, which causes abortion in cattle and undulant fever in humans, has not been positively incriminated as one of the infective agents, but neither has it been completely ruled out.

27. Strangles

Strangles, also called distemper, is caused by a pus-forming organism called the *Streptococcus equi.* It is an infectious and highly contagious disease which can spread like wildfire through a stable or a pasture. It is most likely to affect young horses, but any age is obviously susceptible.

Symptoms

The early symptoms are similar to those of the common cold—lassitude, loss of appetite, elevated temperature, and increased pulse. However, in strangles the nasal discharge appears rapidly, and this very quickly becomes purulent—thick wads of pus running from the nostrils *(photo 1)*.

There is invariably a sore throat, and the horse may have difficulty in swallowing.

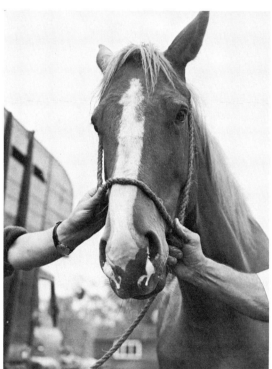

1

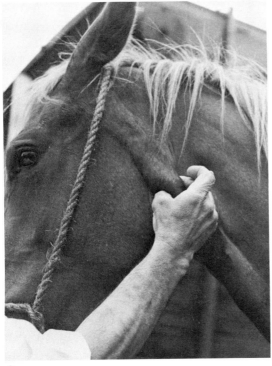

2

Within a few hours the lymph nodes of the head start to swell. The nodes most commonly affected are those between the angles of the lower jaw, but the parotid nodes behind and underneath the ears *(photo 2)* may also be affected.

The nodes swell and are very painful to the touch. Eventually, abscesses form. Sometimes the lymphatic involvement extends to the nodes at the base of the neck, or even into the thorax.

Treatment

With strangles, isolation must be absolute and complete. In addition, all feeding and grooming utensils should be disinfected daily in an iodide solution or a comparable antiseptic, and any bedding removed from the stall should be burned. The horse should have fresh air but be kept comfortably warm and out of drafts.

Those horses which are systemically ill (fever, bad appetite, etc.) will generally be given antibiotics (usually penicillin). Hot compresses applied directly over the involved lymph nodes will encourage the abscess or abscesses   121 to point (drain to the outside.) In some cases the abscesses are opened surgically.

The addition of a soft diet (warm mashes, etc.) will help ease the difficulty in swallowing that is often encountered in these cases.

In the vast majority of cases of strangles, abscesses are confined to the head, but occasionally they may appear on any part of the body where there is a lymph node—the inside or outside of the legs or near the various internal organs, such as the liver or kidneys. In the odd case where this does occur, the horse may die or have to be destroyed. Fortunately, the modern use of antibiotics has made the fatal case of strangles a rarity.

A course of antibiotics is therefore vital, and it is important to start the course as early as possible—at the first sign of symptoms—especially if strangles is known to be in the area.

Prevention

Strangles vaccines are available, but many veterinarians will advise against them (see chapter 6, "Immunization"). The best prevention is to avoid exposure.

THORAX OR CHEST

28. Pneumonia

In the horse, as in all other animals and in humans, pneumonia is brought about by inflammation of the lungs. The usual cause is infection by a virus or bacteria, but fungi may also be a cause.

Mechanical pneumonias can be caused either by direct injury or by fluid that finds its way into the lungs during drenching with a stomach pump.

In virus or bacterial pneumonia, the infection often starts in the lower part of *one* or *both* lungs. The infection spreads from the bottom lobes upwards (see *figure 1*).

As in all other inflammations, there is an initial swelling which blocks up the air spaces that would normally take in the air and oxygen. The swelling is followed by an inflammatory exudate—a fluid discharge—and this closes up still more of the lung spaces.

If large parts of both lungs become affected, the horse is unable to take in sufficient oxygen to keep its heart and body going and death will follow.

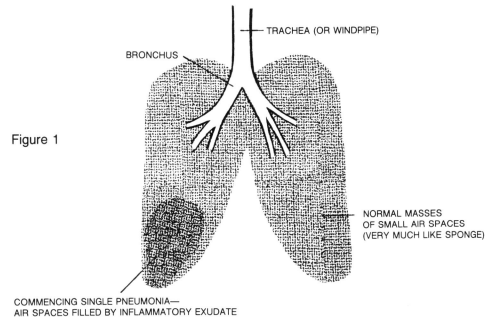

Figure 1

TRACHEA (OR WINDPIPE)

BRONCHUS

NORMAL MASSES
OF SMALL AIR SPACES
(VERY MUCH LIKE SPONGE)

COMMENCING SINGLE PNEUMONIA—
AIR SPACES FILLED BY INFLAMMATORY EXUDATE

125

Symptoms

Symptoms include fever and chill, weakness, diminished appetite, constipation, and rapid shallow breathing. Sometimes nasal discharge is present, sometimes a cough.

Treatment

Immediate skilled veterinary attention is vital, since a prolonged course of a broad-spectrum antibiotic will be necessary to effect a cure. And of course, as in all respiratory infections, good nursing is extremely important.

29. Equine Influenza

This condition occurs all over the world, year round. It has been such a nuisance in the horse world during recent years that I think it best to deal with it on a simple question-and-answer basis.

What Causes It?

The cough *(photo 1),* which is a chief characteristic, is caused by a virus that is related to the human influenza virus, type A.

At What Age Does It Attack?

All ages can be affected, but young foals are particularly susceptible.

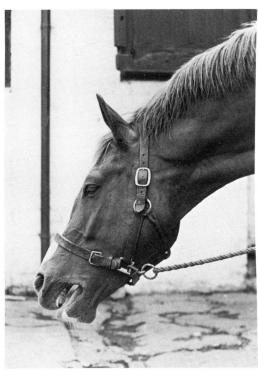

1

Is It Infectious?

Highly so. It sweeps through stables and studs, spreads rapidly throughout an entire district, and can affect 90 to 100 percent of the horses, ponies, and foals.

How Serious Is It?

It is rarely fatal in adults unless untreated complications are allowed to develop. In foals, however, mortality may be high.

Where Does the Virus Strike?

The virus causes an inflammation of the linings of the bronchioles, the small air spaces of the lungs. This explains why the typical case of influenza does not develop a pussy nasal discharge, but only a slight colorless or watery discharge from the nostrils.

How Long Does It Take to Develop?

The incubation period is very short—only a few days.

What Are the Symptoms?

There is an initial fever which rapidly subsides and is often unnoticed. Then the coughing starts, and this is really the only important symptom. The cough is harsh, dry, and painful, many horses becoming markedly distressed. The coughing persists with little or no clear nasal discharge, but neither the eyes nor the lymph nodes are involved. Initially, muscle soreness and marked lethargy are prominent symptoms.

Is There Any Treatment?

Sensible nursing is the main therapy. Stop working the patient immediately and do not start again until the cough has disappeared. This may mean a rest of from several weeks to, occasionally, even several months. Consult your veterinarian immediately regarding the protection of any young susceptible foals.

If the patient should stop eating or appear fevered, your veterinarian will prescribe a course of antibiotic injections to control any secondary pneumonia organisms.

Prevention

Vaccines are available to protect against this disease. They appear at this

time to be quite effective.

30. Pleurisy

The word *pleurisy* simply means an inflammation of the pleura, the fine membrane that lines the chest and covers the lungs. The inflammation is caused by bacteria.

Pleurisy rarely occurs on its own. It comes with, or as a sequel to, various respiratory infections, pneumonia, or strangles.

In the early stages, the pleurisy is usually a "dry" pleurisy; that is, there is no fluid between the two layers of the pleura. Both surfaces (the inside of the

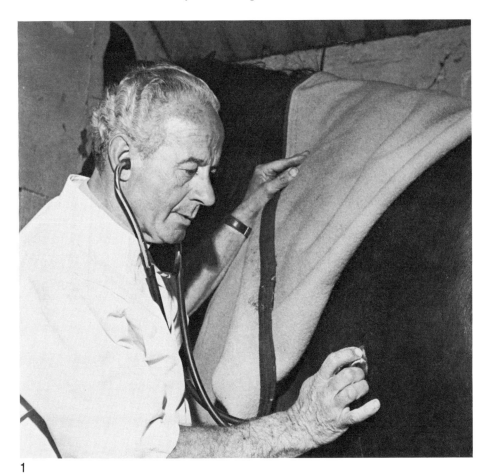

1

part lining the chest wall, and the outside of the part covering the lung) are inflamed and roughened. Obviously, there is considerable pain as the two rough surfaces rub against each other during breathing. Often the pleurisy (pleuritis) is the result of abscessation (abscess formation) within the lung field which breaks into the thoracic cavity.

Symptoms

Breathing is shallow and rapid, and careful examination of the chest with a stethoscope *(photo 1)* reveals dry, rough sounds somewhat like two pieces of sandpaper being rubbed together. This examination, of course, is a job for your veterinarian.

As the case advances, fluid is discharged into the pleural cavity. The pleurisy is now described as a "wet" pleurisy, and an experienced veterinarian will have little difficulty in diagnosing this stage.

Treatment

The veterinarian will prescribe antibiotic therapy. If the pleural fluid is excessive, the horse will have difficulty in breathing and it may be necessary to drain as much fluid as possible. Puncture is effected behind the elbow. In some cases one or several gallons of fluid may have to be drained off. If this is not done, the fluid may cause asphyxia or suffocation by simple pressure on the outside surfaces of the lungs—a pressure that prevents the intake of sufficient air or oxygen.

31. The Horse's Wind

When a horse is sold, it is frequently warranted "sound in wind." This means that the horse's breathing apparatus is in perfect working order.

A sound horse breathes inward and outward through its nostrils, *never* through its mouth; this is anatomically impossible.

The air travels up the nasal passages into the larynx, or voice box, through the trachea, and into the lungs, one on either side of the chest.

The lungs can be likened to two sponges; that is, they are made up of innumerable minute cavities, or spaces.

In these cavities the air, when it fills them, exchanges its oxygen for carbon dioxide which has been brought there by the blood. The blood is revitalized by this essential oxygen.

The oxygenated blood then travels throughout the body to all the muscles and tissues, where it gives off its oxygen and takes in the carbon dioxide.

Obviously the harder a horse works, the more oxygen it requires. When a horse is galloped, its breathing is accelerated and the heart rate rises; that is, the blood is being pumped faster and faster around the circular course to get more and more oxygen to the muscles where the extra energy is required.

High Blowing

When a horse starts to move, you frequently hear a distinct purring noise on expiration—when the horse breathes out. This noise is known as "high blowing" and is caused by a flapping of the false nostril inside the other nostril. It is *not* an unsoundness.

Bridle Noise

Where a keen horse is being held in with his head pulled into his chest and his neck arched *(photo 1),* you may get another expiratory sound rather like roaring but not so pronounced. This is a "bridle noise"—a whistling noise on expiration. Like high blowing, a bridle noise is not an unsoundness.

In fact, both high blowing and bridle noises are minor things that pass off quickly as soon as the horse is put into work and his head and neck are allowed to move freely.

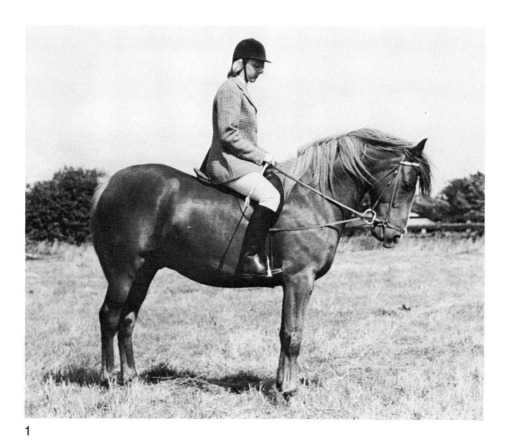

1

Heaves (Broken Wind)

The term *heaves* describes the abnormal breathing pattern encountered in horses with either allergic bronchiolitis or emphysema. Emphysema is usually the result of chronic allergic bronchiolitis. Basically, heaves is an allergic phenomenon resulting from a sensitivity to inhaled particles (dust, pollen, fungal spores, etc.).

As a result of the bronchiolar constriction, it becomes more difficult for the horse not only to bring in sufficient oxygen but to expel air as well. The effort of expiration is so increased that the affected horse makes a two-phase effort; that is, the rib cage closes inward, followed by a contraction of the abdominal musculature to further force out trapped air. With time, and assuming that the problem becomes consistent, the musculature at the lower edge of the rib cage will hypertrophy (overdevelop), and a "heave-line" may appear.

132

Symptoms

The disease is usually first noted by its characteristic deep, nonproductive cough *(photo 2)*. The double expiratory effort and reduced tolerance to exercise are notable signs as well. Seldom is the body temperature elevated above normal. The symptoms (depending on what the individual horse is allergic to) may increase or decrease with the seasons and housing.

Treatment

Ideally, one attempts to remove the allergen or allergens (the cause of the allergic response) from the horse's environment. This is, however, easier said than done, as often the offending particle or particles may be nonremovable. In any case, it is best to get such animals out of a barn or a stable. Medication is helpful and often necessary; unfortunately, for some horses it may become continually necessary and therefore may have long-term ill effects. For this reason every effort should be made to cut down on dust and other particulate matter and to make sure that all enclosures are well ventilated.

In the event that the condition has advanced to emphysema, the terminal air sacs have ruptured and often create large nonfunctional cavities. The damage at this point is irreversible; the lungs will never heal.

Roaring (Laryngeal Hemiplegia)

The larynx *(figure 1)* forms the entrance to the trachea (windpipe). It acts as a valve, opening and closing like two saloon doors. If the nerves which

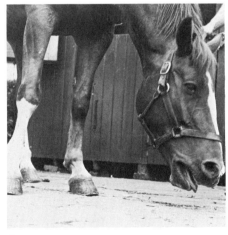

2

Figure 1

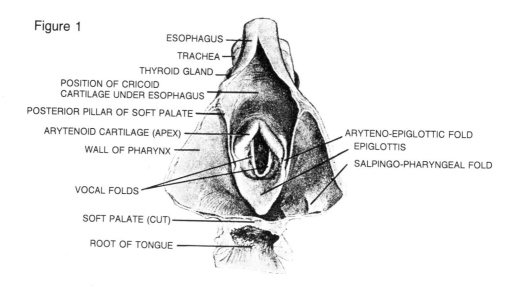

ESOPHAGUS
TRACHEA
THYROID GLAND
POSITION OF CRICOID
CARTILAGE UNDER ESOPHAGUS
POSTERIOR PILLAR OF SOFT PALATE
ARYTENOID CARTILAGE (APEX)
WALL OF PHARYNX
ARYTENO-EPIGLOTTIC FOLD
EPIGLOTTIS
SALPINGO-PHARYNGEAL FOLD
VOCAL FOLDS
SOFT PALATE (CUT)
ROOT OF TONGUE

operate the "doors" are damaged, the larynx becomes paralyzed (one or both sides remain closed). This is usually unilateral (one side), and more often than not on the left side.

The result is an impaired flow of inspired air and the production of an abnormal noise heard on inspiration.

For the most part, this problem is confined to larger, longer-necked horses.

Treatment

Medical therapy is of no known value. Surgical correction is often successful, depending on the degree of paralysis in the individual horse. It should be pointed out, however, that the nerve damage is irreparable.

Tracheotomy

Sometimes called "tubing" (in England), this means surgically inserting a special tube into the horse's windpipe *(photo 3)*. The operation should be performed only by a veterinarian and always under a suitable anesthetic.

A tracheotomy is performed when the upper airway above the tracheotomy site is obstructed (allergic swelling, foreign body, strangles, etc.) in such a way as to require an artificial opening for proper oxygenation.

134

How to Test a Horse's Wind

The following routine has been evolved from a lifetime's experience of examining horses:

1. Check for scars over the windpipe *(photo 4)* and make sure that the skin is free over the larynx or voice box.

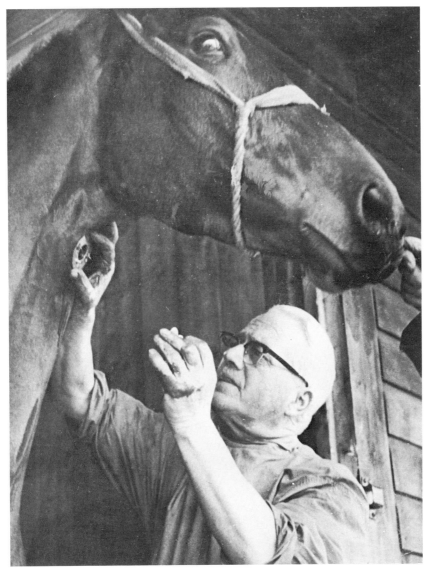

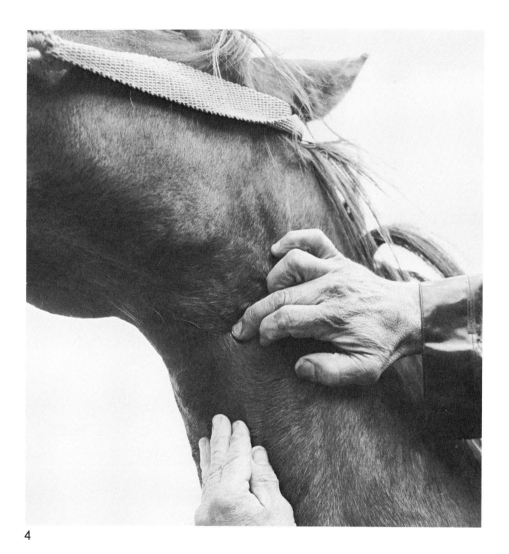

4

2. Watch the horse quietly at rest in his stall; look carefully at his flank for any double expiratory lift.

3. Listen intently, with the ear or with a stethoscope *(photo 5),* to both lungs for any abnormal sounds. Obviously, this has to be done by a veterinarian.

4. Squeeze the horse's larynx with the thumb and forefinger *(photo 6).* If he coughs, be suspicious.

5. Check his pulse and temperature (chapter 7). These should be normal; if elevated, the cough could be caused by a common cold or some other

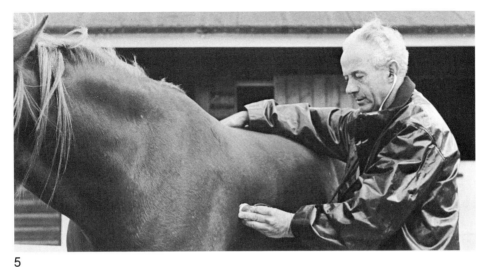

5

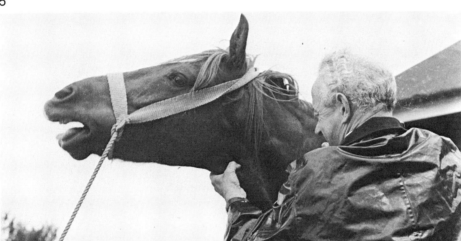

6

infection. If the temperature and/or pulse are in any way abnormal, the horse should not be tested further until he has completely recovered.

6. If the pulse and temperature are normal, put on the saddle and bridle and take him out into the field.

Canter the horse in a small circle on the right rein or, if someone else is riding, stand at the *outside* of the circle so that the horse passes very close and his breathing is clearly audible. Make him do several circles at a slow riding canter. Then put him onto the other rein and repeat the circling.

137

7. If no suspicious noise or distress is spotted, send him on a sharp gallop across the field—fast—for a distance of at least half a mile. When he is pulled up, listen very carefully at his nostrils for any sign of whistling or roaring which, remember, will be heard as he *breathes in.* Also take another look at his flanks and check again for the double lift. Again, this is a point when the veterinarian can listen to the lungs for emphysema.

8. One final point. Always beware when a horse is brought up from grass with a big belly and carrying excess weight ("pigfat"). Often such animals may make noises similar to whistling or roaring. It is much better to go back at a later date to see such a horse, when he is fit or fined down; otherwise, you may wrongly condemn him.

ABDOMEN

32. Colic

Colic is the name given to a symptom, abdominal pain. It is defined as a paroxysm (sudden attack) of griping pain in the abdomen. There are several types:

1. *Flatulent colic.* This is the most common, occurring when there is a collection of gas in the bowel. As it passes through, the gas dilates the bowel abnormally and causes a lot of pain. It is the least serious type of colic, though it is often the most violent.

2. *Obstructive colic.* This occurs when there is a hard mass of food or feces in the bowel that prohibits the passage of all materials (see *figure 1*).

3. *Twist colic.* Here the bowel becomes twisted. This is by far the most serious kind of colic, since it is usually fatal.

All these conditions require immediate veterinary attention, since the seriousness of the condition cannot be judged by the amount of pain the animal shows. The best guide is the pulse, which should beat 40 times per minute. If it rises only slightly, even though the pain is great, the condition is not serious. But if the pulse rises to 80 or 100, it is very serious.

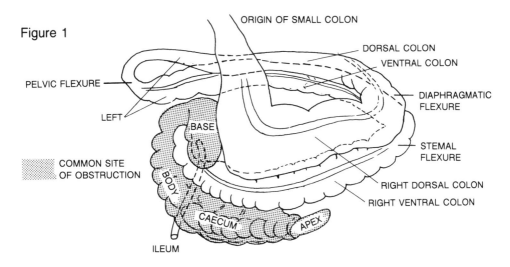

Figure 1

ORIGIN OF SMALL COLON

DORSAL COLON
VENTRAL COLON

PELVIC FLEXURE

DIAPHRAGMATIC FLEXURE

LEFT

BASE

STEMAL FLEXURE

COMMON SITE OF OBSTRUCTION

BODY

RIGHT DORSAL COLON
RIGHT VENTRAL COLON

CAECUM

APEX

ILEUM

First Aid Precautions

Veterinarians' views tend to vary widely on the subject of colic, but most agree that at the first sign of pain all food, including hay, should be removed from the box stall, and the bed made deep and comfortable. A common idea is that the horse should be taken out and kept walking, but in my opinion this is not advisable and is unkind.

Another common belief is that if the horse is allowed to roll, twist of the bowel will occur. I disagree. Horses roll normally and healthily and never twist a bowel, and they will not do it when they have colic. In a twisted gut, the gut is always twisted before the pain starts. The only reason one would want to prevent rolling is that it may become excessive and damaging to other areas—head, neck, legs, etc.

Causes

Most colics result from parasitic problems, but some come from bad management. Common faults include:

Quantity of food. Too little or too much. Ration must be adjusted to work.

Quality of food. Immature or newly thrashed grain. Damaged foods—for example, grain overheated in stack, musty hay, dirty food. Poor-quality roughage, such as chopped straw, oat chaff. Boiled foods may cause abdominal distension.

Irregular feeding. Leads to disordered peristalsis, upsetting the normal contractions that move the food through the intestines. Long intervals between meals result in the horse's gorging food without proper mastication.

Sudden changes in diet. For example, immediate introduction to heavy-concentrate rations or to young, lush pasture.

Watering. Insufficient clean water. Irregular times of watering. Watering when hot, sweating, or exhausted.

Bad work habits. Excessive work, leading to exhaustion; even moderate work, when not in full training. Irregular work, particularly an idle period followed by a long, hard day. Failure to allow cooling-off period on return.

Accidents. Likely to occur when a horse breaks loose and gorges itself on concentrates.

Parasites. Bloodworms (strongylus species) create havoc in the blood vessels supplying the bowel. This can cause obstruction of vessels and thus diminished or occluded blood supply. Roundworms (which occur in young horses) can reach a high enough concentration to block the small bowel.

Anatomic abnormalities. The most common are umbilical and inguinal hernias, the problem being that sections of intestine find themselves entrapped in the hernial sacs.

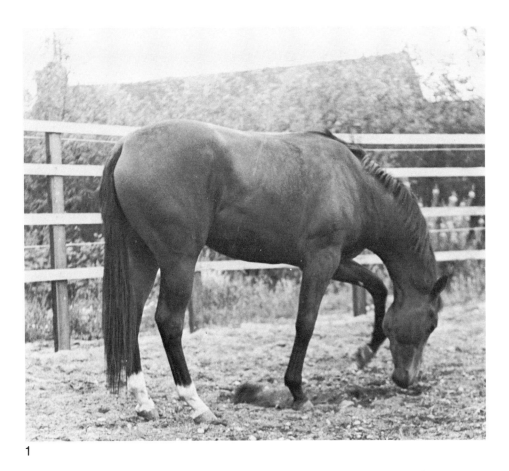

1

Symptoms

Flatulent colic. This is sometimes called spasmodic colic because the accumulation of gas in the bowel causes periodic pain; there will be quiet spells, then violent spells.

The pain in this type of colic is often more extreme than in either of the other two, though the pulse often does not rise to more than about 50.

Obstructive colic. The pain is not so severe but is more consistent, often causing the animal to paw *(photo 1)*.

The pulse may rise a little higher than in flatulent colic (into the 60s). The impaction can frequently, but not always, be felt by a veterinarian in an examination by rectum.

When the veterinarian listens to the abdomen with ear or stethoscope, the absence of sounds of intestinal movement will help diagnose this type of colic. Naturally, if the bowel is impacted, normal movement is inhibited.

143

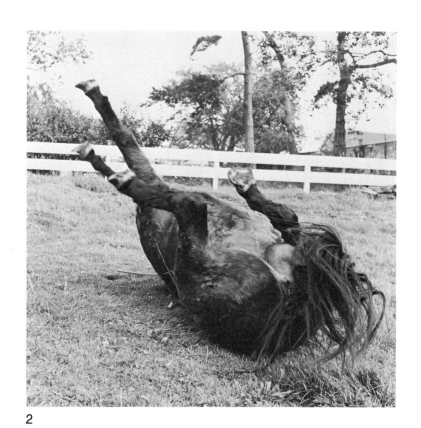

2

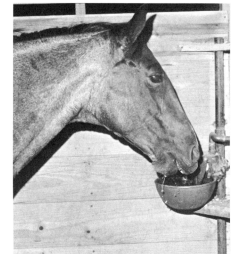

3

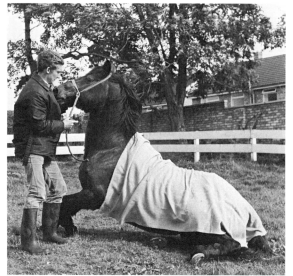

4

Twist Colic. Though usually fatal, in rare instances twist colic may correct itself. Usually the pulse is greatly elevated (80 or more) and the pain is severe and continuous. The horse will often go down and roll. *(photo 2)*. Such horses need immediate attention.

There are, of course, other conditions that can cause colic in horses, such as ruptured stomach, peritonitis, and kidney problems, but these are comparatively uncommon and certainly very much a matter for your veterinarian to diagnose and deal with.

Treatment

As mentioned, colic should always be diagnosed and treated by a veterinarian. So-called "colic drinks" can be purchased, but practically all of them contain a sedative that will mask the symptoms, make the veterinarian's diagnosis much more difficult, and may actually be misleading.

Always confine yourself to the routine first aid described early in this chapter. Modern drugs available include antispasmodics and tranquilizers, both of which help control the pain.

Prevention

Avoid the causes mentioned here. The most important preventives are frequent deworming and correct feeding and watering. Always remember that the horse's stomach is quite small (it normally holds about 2½ gallons and, at a maximum, 4 gallons), so he must be fed in comparatively small quantities at frequent intervals and, most important of all, on a regular schedule. Unlike a mule or a cow, if the horse is allowed to go a long time without food or water, he will attack it greedily when he gets it and upset his digestive rhythm. *Fresh water should be available at all times (photo 3).*

Two further observations on colic:

First, a "doglike" posture is always a bad sign; that is, when the patient sits up like a dog *(photo 4)*, This usually indicates one of the fatal colics resulting from a ruptured stomach or bowel.

Second, renal colic (kidney colic) is not common in the horse, contrary to general opinion. The symptoms are those of abdominal pain, but the pain is not nearly as severe as in the other types of colic. It may be caused by stones blocking the ureter or urethra, and there may or may not be blood in the urine. Diagnosis is difficult and should always be left to the veterinarian, who will no doubt examine the urine in a laboratory.

33. Enteritis

Enteritis simply means inflammation of the bowel or intestinal lining. When this happens, the peristaltic waves that are continually passing along the intestinal wall become accelerated and force the bowel contents along much faster than normal. The glands in the wall of the intestine secrete an excess of fluid; at the same time the intestinal wall does not absorb the usual quantity of fluid because it doesn't get the time or the chance. The result produces the typical signs of enteritis.

Symptoms

In the acute stages, spasmodic pain and diarrhea; this may be copious, so much so that the horse may appear to pass nothing more or less than hot water *(photo 1).*

Causes

These are varied. They may be:

Bacterial.

Dietetic. The animal may have eaten, for example, moldy hay, bran, or oats, all of which may contain fungi that can cause a very acute enteritis.

Chemical. Lead from chewing paint, for example.

Vegetable. Certain poisonous plants may have been eaten during grazing.

Unknown. One of the most severe and often fatal forms of enteritis in the horse is a disease referred to as Colitis X. Its cause is unknown. It usually follows a stressful situation (shipping, racing, showing, etc.).

Treatment

Enteritis can be one of the most serious of all equine complaints, so send for your veterinarian at once. Never try "do-it-yourself" treatments on a horse with diarrhea.

If the patient is on pasture, bring him up into a warm stall, blanket him, and leave the diagnosis and treatment to your veterinarian, whose first concern will be to try to establish the cause. Having done so, the veterinarian will then prescribe antispasmodics, sedatives, and possibly antibiotics, and attempt to restore what is being lost (water, electrolytes, etc.).

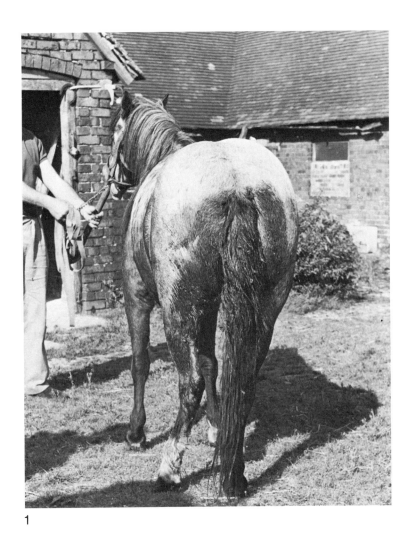

1

Never give purgatives. They may produce a fatal superpurgation or dysentery. As in all animals, the horse is susceptible to dehydration (loss of body fluids), which can in itself cause death. It may well be necessary for your veterinarian to inject fluid intravenously in the form of normal saline solution or a multiple electrolyte solution.

Follow-up Treatment

When the patient is recovering and convalescent, he should be put very gradually onto food. Bran mashes are undoubtedly the best to begin with—three a day for at least three days.

34. Nephritis

Kidney inflammation, called nephritis, is comparatively uncommon in the young horse, but it is my experience that chronic nephritis often occurs in horses and ponies from the age of fifteen or sixteen years onward. The condition is more common in mares than in geldings, especially if they have been used for breeding. The patient in *photo 1* was just over twenty years old.

Nephritis also shows up sometimes in horses that are allowed to graze on sorghum, sorghum hybrids, or even Johnson grass, which is related to sorghum.

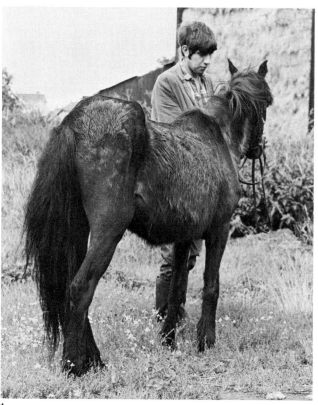

1

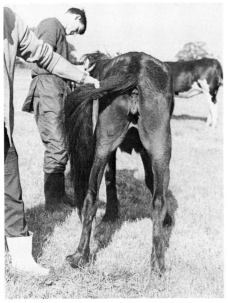

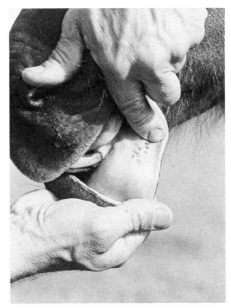

2   3

Symptoms

Progressive loss in condition, despite a good appetite, and deposits around the vulva (*photo 2*) or penis may occur. Many owners repeatedly treat such cases for worms with, of course, no success whatsoever.

The reason the affected horse becomes emaciated is that protein (which should be used to repair and build up muscles and tissues) is excreted through the damaged kidneys into the urine instead of being passed to the liver for the body's utilization. After a few weeks, well-marked ulcers often appear in the mouth (*photo 3*).

Treatment

Send for your veterinarian. He or she will take blood and urine samples, assess the amount of damage, and prescribe treatment if at all possible.

It is my experience that chronic nephritis cases rarely respond to treatment; sooner or later the patient goes down and is unable to rise. Euthanasia may be indicated.

LEGS

35. Lameness

Lameness is generally an indication of pain in one or more legs. There is, however, one other type of lameness—mechanical lameness. This arises when there is a stiffness in a joint or a contraction of a tendon whereby, mechanically, the horse is unable to move his leg in a normal manner. He is definitely lame though suffering no pain.

With most lamenesses involving limb pain, one must first establish which limb or limbs are involved. At times this is difficult, but with practice and close observation it becomes easier. First, watch the horse at a walk, away from you and then back toward your line of vision. If the problem is severe enough, it will be apparent at the walk. Often the horse will raise or nod his head when the affected *forelimb* contacts the ground (this helps to take the weight off the affected limb). One will often detect a difference in sound, since the involved limb does not contact the ground as hard as the normal limbs.

It is best to compare the swing and the landing position of the front legs and then repeat the same visualization with the hind legs. Usually all views—from front, back, and sides—are necessary to be sure which limb is involved. This is best accomplished on a hard, flat surface. The horse should be trotted as well *(photo 1);* you often find that the lameness will be more obvious when the horse is trotted in a circle. The canter and gallop are not very helpful; lameness becomes difficult to discern because of the relative speed the moving limbs attain.

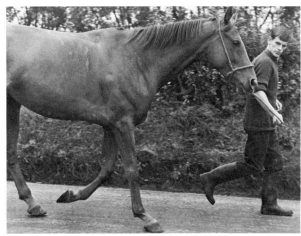

1

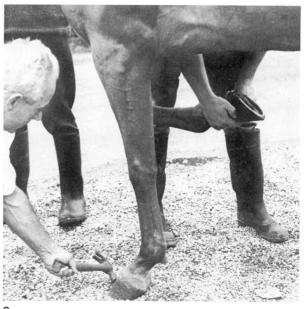

2

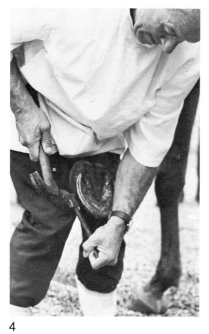

4

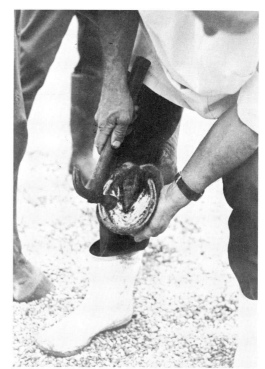

3

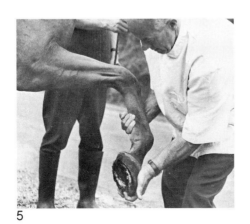

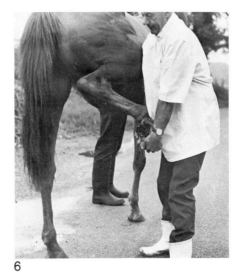

5

6

Examining the Individual Leg for Lameness

Always start at the foot and always examine the foot, no matter where you think the lameness may be. Have the sound leg lifted and tap the suspect foot all around with a hammer *(photo 2)*.

Then let the other forefoot down; lift the affected one and tap all around the sole *(photo 3)*. If the horse evinces any pain, call your veterinarian immediately. He or she may wish to have the shoe removed (or remove it in person, *(photo 4)* and will search the foot carefully for a picked-up nail, a puncture, an abscess, a bruise, etc.

If there is no sign of pain in the foot, start at the coronet and work up gradually, looking for any sign of swelling, pain, or abnormality.

The fetlock joint should be put into complete flexion and held that way for some time *(photo 5);* then the horse should be trotted again. If the lameness is more marked, the joint surface is probably involved. If there is no result, repeat in turn with the knee, the elbow, and the shoulder.

With a hind-leg lameness, follow the same procedure *(photo 6)*. Unfortunately, however, it is impossible to bend the hock without bending the stifle, and this makes it extremely difficult to differentiate between a hock and a stifle lameness.

Obviously, the diagnosis of lameness requires a great deal of skill and experience and is indeed a job for the veterinarian. Nonetheless, by following the simple rules I have given, it is possible to make an intelligent guess as to the location, if not the cause, of the lameness, to be subsequently confirmed and investigated by the professional.

155

36. Spavin

Spavin is the common name given to a degenerative arthrosis (arthritis) of the lower joints of the hock. Usually it may appear as a hard, bony swelling (similar to a ringbone) or callosity which occurs at the front, inside, and lower edge of the hock joint *(photo 1)*. It involves the lower joints of the tarsus and the head of the metatarsus and may be the result of (1) strain or sprain or (2) direct trauma or injury, either of which can cause an inflammation on the surface of the bone which leads to a new growth of bone—an *exostosis*. Often the damage encroaches on the joint surface, producing an arthritis.

Symptoms

The hard, bony swelling is usually accompanied by a chronic or recurrent lameness. This lameness is accentuated when the hock is flexed for thirty to sixty seconds.

Treatment

1. *Complete rest.* As in all inflammations and sprains, rest is far and away the most important factor in healing.

2. *Point firing and blistering* after varying periods of rest. This technique —applying a hot iron or acid to the trouble spot under local anesthesia to create a burn—is controversial. It does have the effect of changing a chronic condition to an acute one. This increases blood circulation and causes other natural body defenses to go to work there. The main object in firing is to enforce rest, but it also assists in the full formation of the callosity or exostosis.

3. More often than not, spavin responds to *anti-inflammatory drugs,* such as Butazolidin, and corrective shoeing. This will depend on the degree of involvement and conformation.

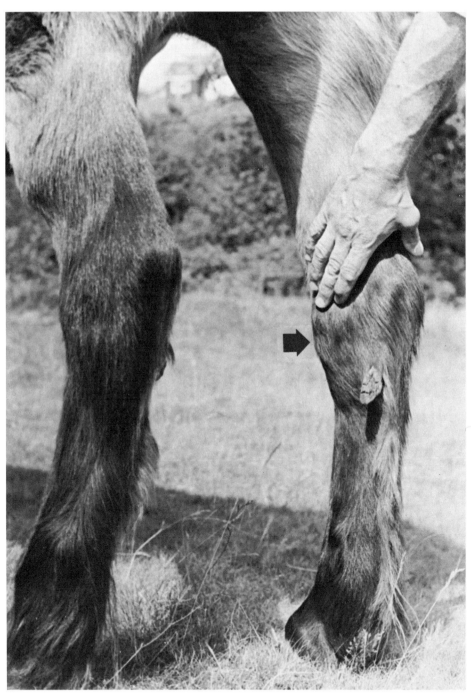

1

37. Ringbone

Ringbone is the common name given to bony change involving the pastern and coffin joints. "High ringbone" refers to change involving the pastern joint, and "low ringbone" refers to the coffin joint *(photos 1* and *2)*.

There are also "articular" and "nonarticular" ringbones. "Articular" simply means that the ringbone involves the *joint*—either between the first and second phalanx or between the second and third phalanx—that is, the joint at the top of the hoof *(photo 3)*. (The third phalanx is the bone of the hoof, the coffin bone.) Nonarticular ringbone develops on the bone—the first or second phalanx—without impinging on the joint.

Ringbone may occur at any age. It is occasionally seen in young horses, but it is more likely to occur in older horses. Heredity, conformation defects, and improper foot balance and shoeing are all predisposing factors. It is caused by trauma (direct injury), by concussion (constant banging on hard roads), or by hereditary predisposition (conformation).

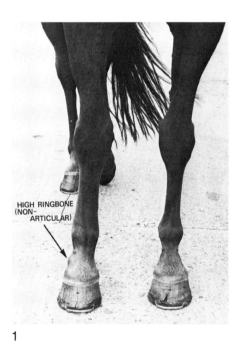

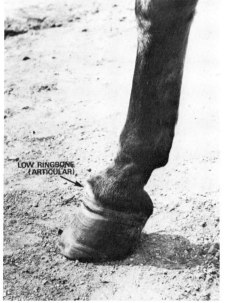

1

2

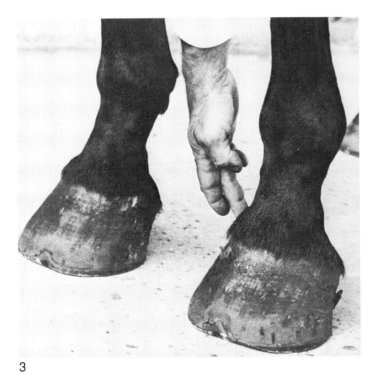

3

Symptoms

The degree of lameness varies and is often (but not always) accompanied by a bony swelling. After a varying period of time of up to several months, the pain on palpation may vanish and the original problem—lameness—lessen or disappear.

Prognosis

In nonarticular lameness, when the callosity or bone is completely formed, the lameness will go, and the chances are that it will not return.

In articular ringbone, however, the prognosis is very grave, and lameness may be permanent.

Treatment

In the first instance, the horse needs complete rest for periods of up to an entire season.

Later, if lameness still persists, firing and blistering may be tried (see chapter 36, "Spavin"), though in articular ringbone there is very little chance of complete success. Corrective shoeing may be helpful in selected cases.

159

38. Splints

In order to understand exactly what splints are, one must understand the anatomy of the metacarpus, or cannon bone, which runs from the knee to the fetlock.

At the back of the cannon bone and to each side of it lie two small metacarpal bones, or "splint bones." They are broad at the top, where they form part of the knee joint, and taper to a point about two thirds of the way down the cannon bone (see *figure 1,* showing the rear view).

Each of these two "splint bones" is attached to the periosteum, or covering of the cannon bone, by a ligament. When there is any excess stress or strain on the forelegs, one or the other of the ligaments may become stretched or sprained, and when this happens the periosteum is pulled away from the bone.

The resultant inflammation causes swelling, local pain, and often marked lameness. The pain and lameness will pass off in two or three weeks, but the swelling will become harder, simply because the inflammatory fluid and tissue change into bone. In doing so, they unite the splint bone directly to the cannon bone.

Commonest Position

The commonest position for splints is the inside splint bone at the junction of the upper third and lower two thirds *(photo 1).*

More Serious Positions

The splint may form on the inside of the splint bone, and it can then be serious. Its presence, even after it has settled down, may interfere with the action of the suspensory and check ligaments which run down the back of the cannon bone between the two splint bones.

When an extensive splint forms across the back of the cannon bone underneath the suspensory ligament, it is sometimes referred to as a blind splint *(figure 2).* Its presence may interfere with the suspensory ligament. When the splint forms at the head of the splint bone, it may interfere with the action of the knee joint. This is called a jack splint. In the event of excessive pain and/or swelling, one may suspect splint bone fracture. Radiographs (x-rays) are necessary to confirm such a diagnosis.

160

Figure 1

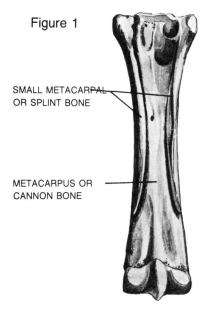

SMALL METACARPAL
OR SPLINT BONE

METACARPUS OR
CANNON BONE

Rear view of cannon bone

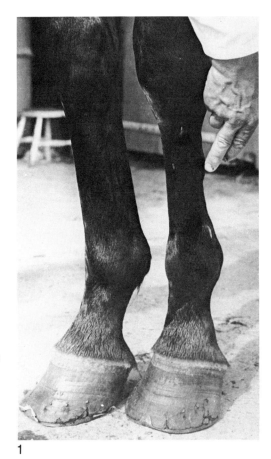

1

Figure 2

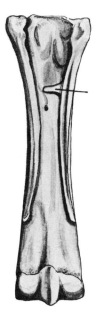

ROD SPLINT EXTENDING UNDER
THE SUSPENSORY LIGAMENT

When They Occur

Splints most frequently appear in young horses (three to four years old) when they start serious work *(photo 2)*.

Symptoms

Lameness. Swelling and pain on pressure over the spot where the splint is developing.

Treatment

Rest is essential until the lameness is gone. This can take up to three or even four weeks.

During the first week of the rest period, poultices may be applied to the part twice daily *(photo 3)*. Your veterinarian will advise on what to use.

A slightly more spectacular treatment comprises injections of cortisone into the swelling, while many veterinarians pin their faith on blistering or point firing and blistering. (See chapter 36, "Spavin").

It is my opinion that poulticing and rest are adequate. They are certainly logical and sensible because time, and time alone, heals satisfactorily. One has to wait until the bone callosity is completely formed.

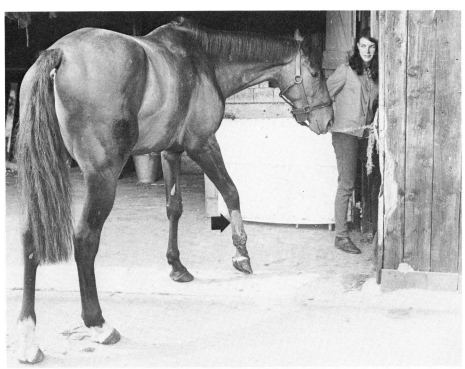

2

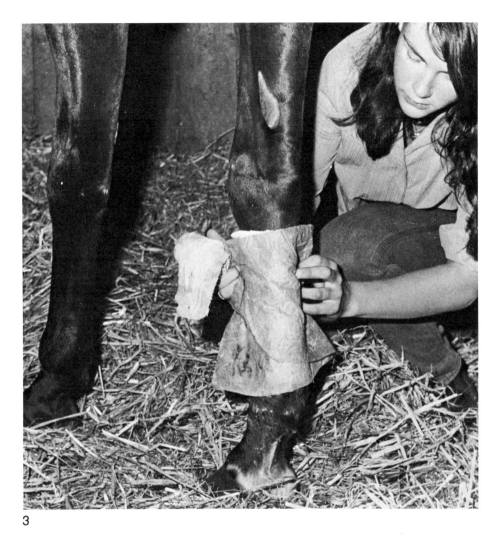

3

After the lameness disappears, work must be introduced only very gradually; otherwise the ligament may tear again and set back the convalescence another month.

Are Splints an Unsoundness?

The average splint is not a serious condition, but it can, and does, spoil the look of a show animal, and some judges will downgrade the affected horse or pony immediately.

Technically speaking, however, a splint does not comprise a major unsoundness unless it involves the suspensory ligament or is fractured.

163

39. Sprained Flexor Tendons

Running down the back of the cannon bones are the two flexor tendons—the superficial and the deep (see *figure 1*). Their function is to bend the legs when the muscles at their upper ends contract.

When the horse is galloping or jumping and extending his legs forward as far as they will go, he puts an immense strain on the flexor tendons each time his forefeet land *(photo 1)*. Frequently, some of the fibers of the tendon give way or, in an extreme case, the whole tendon may rupture. (Also strained is the suspensory ligament—see chapter 43.)

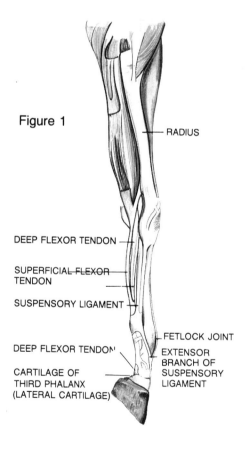

Figure 1

RADIUS

DEEP FLEXOR TENDON

SUPERFICIAL FLEXOR TENDON

SUSPENSORY LIGAMENT

FETLOCK JOINT

DEEP FLEXOR TENDON

EXTENSOR BRANCH OF SUSPENSORY LIGAMENT

CARTILAGE OF THIRD PHALANX (LATERAL CARTILAGE)

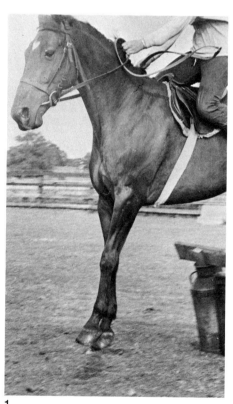

1

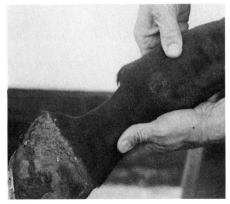

2

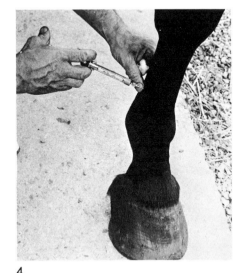

4

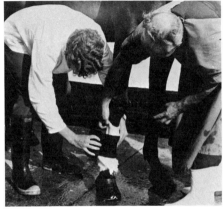

3

Symptoms

In the average case, where only part of one tendon is involved, the usual symptoms are marked lameness, swelling and puffiness over the affected part, and marked pain to the touch *(photo 2)*.

Treatment

Complete rest for a long period is necessary—usually at least for the remainder of the season and certainly for a minimum of three months. In the early stages your veterinarian may advise twice-daily poulticing and bandaging *(photo 3)* or may recommend ice packs, cold-water whirlpools, or similar forms of treatment. He or she may aspirate the fluid (draw it off through a needle), if swelling is excessive, and possibly inject cortisone into the area *(photo 4)*. Opinions as to the best treatment vary.

165

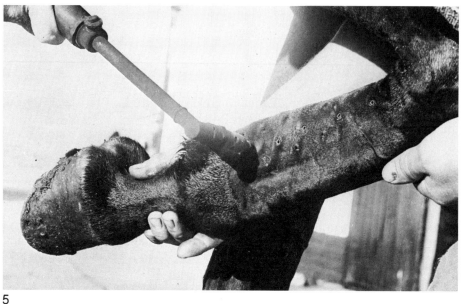

5

If the tendons and suspensory ligament are completely ruptured, the fetlock will be on the ground. Such cases are usually hopeless, but the horse can occasionally be saved for breeding purposes, etc.

After the pain has completely subsided, firing and blistering may be resorted to *(photo 5)*. For some reason this rather drastic treatment often seems to be successful despite the fact that many veterinarians are opposed to it. Perhaps the success of the treatment can be credited mainly to the enforced prolonged rest.

There are numerous methods of firing—line, point, or acid-firing—and the efficacy of each method is debatable. Usually the tendon or ligament that has once been strained is never as strong as it once was and is likely to break down with work.

40. Synovial Distensions

Synovia is a fluid that is produced by synovial membranes, which line the inside of the joints. In addition, they line the sheaths which fit around the tendons, and also numerous small pockets or sacs in various parts of the body—sacs that are called *bursae.*

The synovia acts as a lubricant to keep the joints working smoothly, to keep the tendons moving smoothly in their sheaths, and to lubricate the bursae so that they may satisfactorily glide either over a point of bone or around a corner.

If, for any reason, the synovial membrane becomes inflamed in part or in whole, it will release more than the normal quantity of fluid into the joint, tendon sheath, or bursa, and a swelling—usually not painful—will result. Such a swelling is known as a synovial distension *(photo 1).*

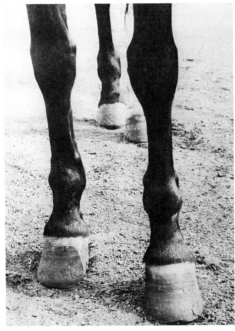

1

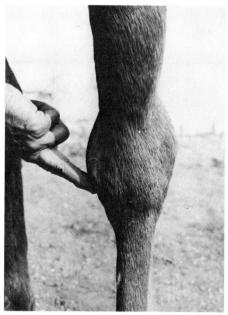 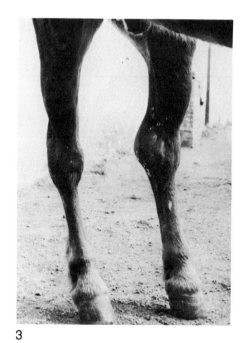

2   3

Bog Spavin

This is a synovial swelling that appears on the inside of the hock toward the front, but higher than the site of ordinary spavin *(photo 2)*. The swelling is soft and not painful. A bog spavin usually represents a cosmetic rather than a lameness problem.

Treatment

If no lameness is present, it is best to leave well enough alone.

Boggy Hock

A boggy hock is basically the same situation as a bog spavin, the differences being that it involves the whole joint capsule and that the swelling is uniform around the hock *(photo 3)*. Again, it is not painful.

Boggy hock frequently occurs in young horses on pasture. Usually, however, when they are brought up and put to work, the swelling disappears.

In old horses, unfortunately, the swelling may not disappear, and in most cases it becomes permanent.

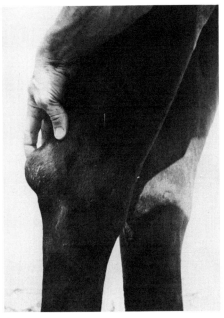

4

A boggy hock is usually considered an unsoundness, even though it is not ordinarily associated with lameness.

Treatment

If the horse is not lame, leave it alone; if he is lame, send for your veterinarian.

Capped Hock

At the point of the hock there is a bursa; this occasionally becomes enlarged and filled with fluid. When it does, it is known as a capped hock *(photo 4)*.

An injury causes capped hock: it is produced perhaps by the horse's kicking at a stable wall or at any hard object or perhaps by repeated knocking on a hard or slippery stable or loose stall floor in attempts to get up.

In the early stages, since it is the result of an injury, it is painful because of the general bruising, but the fluid in the bursa does not give rise to pain, though it usually persists and leaves some permanent swelling.

Capped hock is not an unsoundness, however, though it must be mentioned on a veterinary certificate.

Treatment

When it first happens, the cold hose (running water, for ten to twenty minutes) twice daily is as good a treatment as any, but after the pain has subsided, it is futile to apply any treatment, especially since capped hock is not an unsoundness but only a blemish.

Thoroughpin

Just above the hock, both on the inside and on the outside and to the back of the hock, run two tendon sheaths. These frequently become distended with synovial fluid, and the resultant swelling is known as a thoroughpin *(photo 5)*.

Like capped hock, a thoroughpin is only a blemish, not an unsoundness, and, again, the best treatment is to leave well enough alone.

Windgalls (Windpuffs)

Above the fetlocks, on the inside and on the outside, are two tendon sheaths. When these become filled and dilated with synovial fluid, they produce the condition known as windgalls, or windpuffs *(photo 6)*.

Windgalls occur most frequently in older horses and can affect both the fore and the hind legs. They may be an unsightly blemish, but they are not classified as an unsoundness.

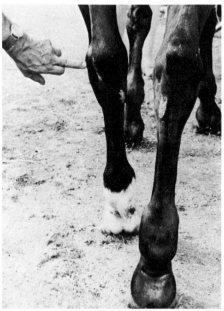
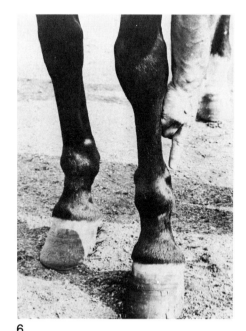

5   6

Capped Elbow

On the point of the elbow there is another bursa. Certain horses or ponies, when getting up or down, strike the point of the elbow with the heel of their fore shoe. This produces a synovial swelling within the bursa and gives rise to the condition called a capped elbow or an elbow gall *(photo 7).*

The way to prevent capped elbow is to keep the feet regularly shod, with the heels not too long *(photo 8).*

General Treatment of Synovial Distensions

Treatment of any or all synovial distensions is not of much avail, except in the early inflammatory stages (see under "Capped Hock").

The distensions can be aspirated (the fluid drawn off with a needle) and injected with various preparations, the most popular being cortisone injected into the joint.

However, since the capsule of the distension still remains, nature will rapidly fill it up and the condition will return.

The best advice, therefore, is generally to take no action and learn to live with the blemish. In the case of a capped elbow, if the problem continues to increase, a "shoe-boil" roll is often used. This is nothing more than a thick bandage applied around the pastern to prevent contact of the heel of the shoe with the elbow.

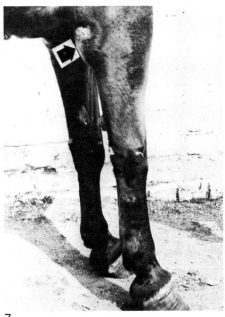

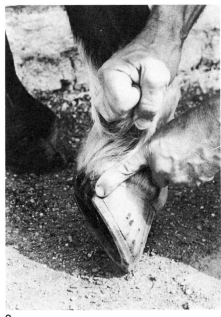

7
8

171

41. Fractures

Fractures may involve any bone or bones. Obviously, the future of such a problem is dependent on the type of fracture, the location of the fracture, the age and size of the horse, and, to a great degree, the temperament of the animal. Recent advances in equine orthopedic surgery have increased the likelihood of saving horses that in the past would have been destroyed. Saving them, however, requires a large investment of both money and time.

There is one type of fracture that can be treated successfully and comparatively inexpensively—a fracture without displacement *(photo 1)*. Such a break should always be suspected when a horse has been kicked on the legs by another horse, especially when the kicker is shod. It is sometimes called a "star" fracture, and in most cases it can be diagnosed only by x-ray *(photo 2)*. It is always advisable, therefore, to have a kicked leg x-rayed as quickly as possible. If the fracture is missed, it may displace later, producing a compound break which will probably be irreparable.

Treatment

Fractures are obviously very much a job for your veterinarian, who will most likely fit a plaster cast *(photo 3)*. The patient may have to be slung (his body partially supported by slings designed for the purpose) and will certainly require at least six months' rest. Because of the enforced inactivity, the diet will have to be adjusted.

The prognosis will vary with the location of the break, the degree of displacement and associated tissue damage, and other variables which affect the horse.

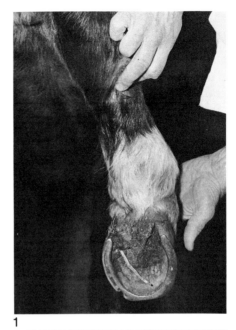

1

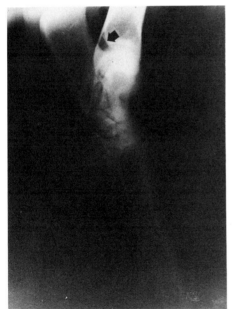

2

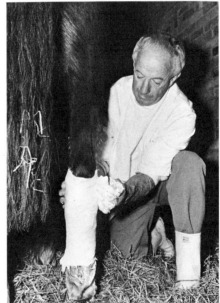

3

42. Curb

At the back of the hock there is a strong fibrous ligament which starts just below the point of the hock and runs down to the head of the metatarsus, or cannon bone. The function of this ligament *(plantar ligament)* is to provide support and stability to the back of the hock.

In young horses, this ligament may become strained while the horse is galloping or jumping. The strain is especially likely to happen in horses with bad conformation; for example, sickle hocks—that is, hocks abnormally curved with the foot too far under the body. It is also very common in Standardbred racehorses.

When the ligament is strained or torn, the resultant swelling is called a *curb (photo 1)*. The cause is usually overwork or excessive, violent flexion of the hock.

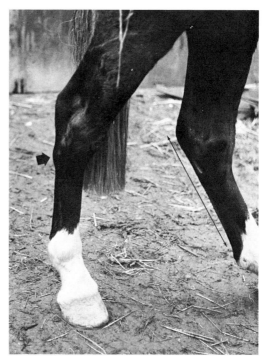

1

Symptoms

In the early stages there is, besides the swelling, considerable pain and a varying degree of lameness. After two or three weeks the lameness and pain will subside, but the swelling or thickening remains. This thickening can be seen by standing back, or it can be felt by running the hand or the tips of the fingers from the point of the hock down the midline at the back.

Treatment

Complete rest is needed, for at least two weeks, and running cold water on the part for five minutes, two or three times daily. *Don't* use liniments or blister, and if in the slightest doubt, consult your veterinarian immediately.

If, at the end of fourteen days, the horse is sound, he may be put into quiet light work, but there should be no heavy work for at least three months. Overwork should be avoided at all times.

Is Curb an Unsoundness?

The answer is yes. Curb does, however, normally stand up better than other ligament strains.

43. Sprain
of the Suspensory Ligament

Sprain (or strain) of the suspensory ligament is reasonably common in hard-working horses (racing, three-day eventing, etc.). When it does happen, the part affected is usually the lower portion where the ligament branches near the fetlock *(photo 1)*.

The suspensory ligaments are elastic ligaments which are involved in the support of the fetlock joint. Sprain, or in some cases complete rupture, can occur during fast galloping or jumping if the horse slips—the primary cause of this injury.

Symptoms

There will be acute lameness and heat and pain immediately above the fetlock. If the ligament is ruptured, the fetlock will tend to drop down below its normal level even though it is still held by the superficial flexor tendon. Any injury to the suspensory ligament is serious and can take a long time to heal.

Treatment

Prolonged rest is necessary usually for at least the remainder of the season.

If the ligament branches are ruptured, the fetlock must be supported either by elastic bandages or, in extreme cases, by a plaster cast.

Prognosis

A mild sprain often responds to long rest and usually heals sufficiently for the horse to be raced again. However, if the ligament is ruptured, complete healing is rare and treatment should be considered only in a mare or a stallion which can be kept for breeding or stud.

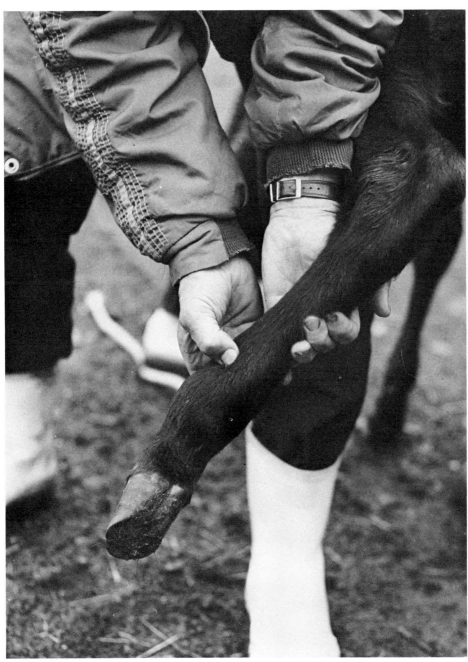

1

44. Stringhalt

The particular problem of stringhalt is poorly understood. It is caused by an excessive flexion of the hock, which produces an upward jerking of one or both hind legs. This is seen either when the horse walks or when he is turned sharply in a small circle *(photo 1)*.

Stringhalt is not a painful condition and does not cause lameness. Nonetheless, it is unsightly and constitutes a definite technical unsoundness.

Many stringhalted horses are serviceable and gallop and jump perfectly satisfactorily. In fact, a stringhalted mare won the British Grand National several years ago.

Treatment

The problem (if excessive) can be treated surgically. The success, however, is variable.

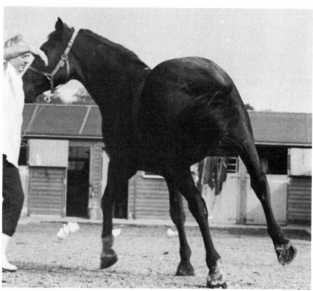

1

45. Shivering

Shivering is an unusual disease whose cause is at present unknown. It is marked by the involuntary shaking of certain groups of muscles, generally in the hind legs but occasionally in the forelegs.

When an affected animal is set or pushed backward, the tail rises and also shivers *(photo 1)*. During shoeing the symptoms may be exaggerated, especially when the shoe is being nailed on. The leg is pushed outward, the shivering increases violently, and the horse may almost fall onto his other side.

A drink of cold water, or cold water thrown over a suspected leg, will often make the symptoms more pronounced.

Treatment

There is no known cure for shivering, but it may disappear.

Is It an Unsoundness?

Yes, shivering is an unsoundness, although, like stringhalt, it is not a painful condition. Also, as with stringhalt, the shivering may get worse with age, unless the horse recovers spontaneously.

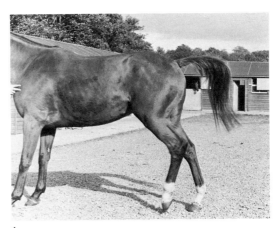

1

46. Lymphangitis

Sporadic lymphangitis (weed, or bigleg) is a condition which generally affects horses that are being fed heavily and worked hard. It flares up when they have to stop their active exercise suddenly—for instance, during spells of snow or frost. It is likely to occur, therefore, in hunters and in hardworking horses.

Symptoms

The patient runs a high temperature—up to 105 or 106 degrees F.—and has an elevated pulse. There is a definite and often severe lameness of one leg, usually a hind leg but occasionally a foreleg.

The lymphatics (the vertical drainage vessels in the legs) become swollen and feel like hard pencils with swollen nodules along their course *(photo 1)*.

Usually, when the swelling starts to appear, the pulse and temperature both drop to near normal despite the fact that the entire leg may continue to swell, sometimes to almost twice the normal size.

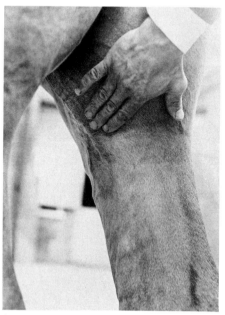

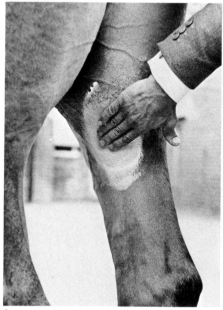

1

2

Treatment

If the diagnosis is certain, massage the swollen lymphatics with an ointment or an oily liquid *(photo 2)*. Continue the massage three or four times daily, and combine each session with a half hour of forced exercise, provided, of course, that the patient is fit to walk. Gentle exercise helps get the lymphatics flowing freely again.

A laxative or a light purgative will be given by your veterinarian, and also, probably, a course of antibiotic injections to prevent secondary infection.

Prevention

When the horse is not at work, his feed should be very much reduced and the oats cut out entirely. Prompt attention to all wounds of the lower extremities and maintenance of a dry stable also help prevent this condition, as well as others. Be aware that it is likely to return.

Other Types of Lymphangitis

Sporadic lymphangitis has been discussed at length because its occurrence hints at lapses in good management. However, the horseman must not be too quick to diagnose it, as it can be confused with other, more sinister, forms of lymphangitis that may require different treatment. There are bacterial and fungal forms of lymphangitis to be considered, especially if wounds or sores are evident, in which case the massage part of the treatment could be detrimental to the horse as well as dangerous to the horseman, since horse and man share susceptibility to many types of infections.

47. Azoturia

Like lymphangitis, azoturia, or Monday morning disease, is a condition following idleness in fit horses. It occurs in hunters and racehorses that have had to be laid off work, usually because of the weather.

Symptoms

When exercise is started after the idle period, the animal will appear perfectly normal and may go for ten to thirty minutes before any signs are noticed. Stiffness is usually the first sign, followed by sweating and obvious signs of pain.

The urine, if and when the patient voids, is coffee-colored or reddish-brown, often described as "wine-colored."

Treatment

On no account must you attempt to walk the horse home. If you do, he will get progressively worse and may eventually go down and possibly die.

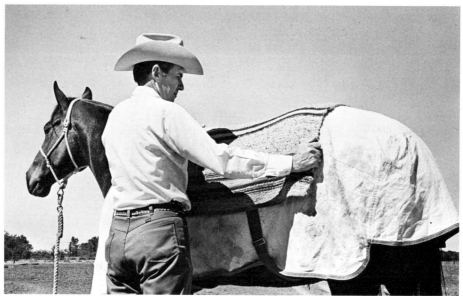

Take him back to his stall in a trailer, if traveling far, and send for your veterinarian at once. He or she will inject antihistamine, cortisone, or Butazolidin and will order complete rest on a restricted diet.

There will be pain in the muscles of the loins, but this will soon pass off with modern treatment. Nonetheless, the old-fashioned treatment of hot blankets across the loins also helps considerably *(photo 1)*.

Treated sensibly and promptly, most horses recover completely. If treatment is delayed, or if the horse is forced to continue after the onset of symptoms, death or permanent kidney damage may result.

If, after a day or two, the horse seems back to normal, exercise can be resumed, but this must be done very gently and very slowly. There is an old saying that still very much applies: "When a horse is being exercised—walk the first mile, trot the next, and do what the hell you like after that."

Prevention

When the horse is not at exercise, drastically reduce his feed and cut oats out entirely.

48. Grease

Grease is an inflammation of the skin on the back part of the pasterns, fetlocks, and lower cannons. Once common on draft horses, it is now seldom seen, and then only on heavier horses. However, it is very common in horses pastured on continually wet grass. It can be likened to diaper rash in infants.

Symptoms

The term grease vividly describes the condition. The leg (usually one but sometimes both hind legs, as shown in *photo 1*) swells up and exudes a foul-smelling greasy discharge. Lameness is not usually present except when the condition is complicated by infection.

Treatment

Stop feeding horse cubes, oats, or linseed—give only good hay and a bran mash twice daily. Get the animal into regular work and house in a roomy box stall.

Wash with soap and water, dry thoroughly, and apply a lotion comprising ½ ounce zinc sulfate, ¼ ounce lead acetate, and 1½ pints water.

If infection is present, an antibiotic aerosol containing chloramphenicol and gentian violet is a useful dressing. Some horses violently resent aerosols. In such cases, the antibiotics have to be applied in lotion form.

Prevention

Feed strictly according to work done and never keep a heavyweight hunter standing idle in a stable.

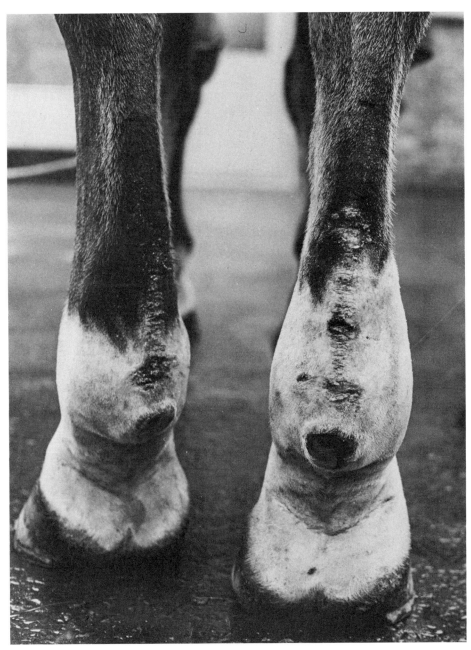

1

FEET

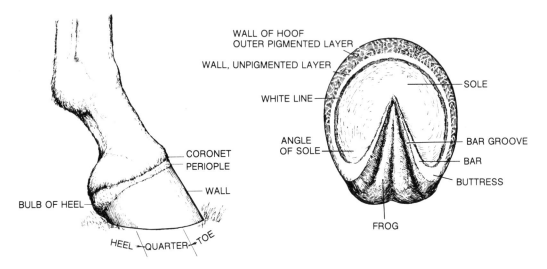

WALL OF HOOF
OUTER PIGMENTED LAYER

WALL, UNPIGMENTED LAYER

WHITE LINE

ANGLE
OF SOLE

SOLE

BAR GROOVE

BAR

BUTTRESS

FROG

CORONET
PERIOPLE

WALL

BULB OF HEEL

HEEL QUARTER TOE

Figure 1

Figure 2

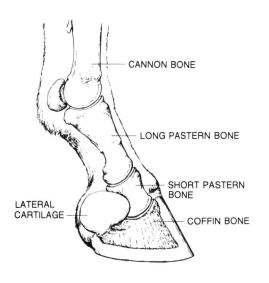

CANNON BONE

LONG PASTERN BONE

SHORT PASTERN
BONE

LATERAL
CARTILAGE

COFFIN BONE

Figure 3

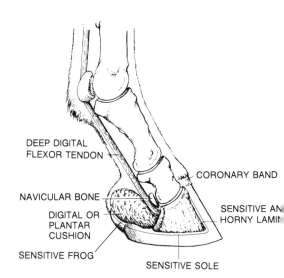

DEEP DIGITAL
FLEXOR TENDON

CORONARY BAND

NAVICULAR BONE

DIGITAL OR
PLANTAR
CUSHION

SENSITIVE AN
HORNY LAMIN

SENSITIVE FROG

SENSITIVE SOLE

Figure 4

49. The Horse's Foot: General Anatomy

A simple knowledge of the anatomy of the horse's foot helps in understanding the need for care and also the various problems that can arise. *Figures 1* and *2* identify the visible parts of the hoof. *Figures 3* and *4* show the main internal structures.

The External Parts

The *coronet* is the upper encircling border of the hoof's horny wall, where hair growth stops. The *wall,* made up of straight fibers growing downward and forward, grows much like the human fingernail and is insensitive except at its very top. Below the coronet is the *periople*—something like the human cuticle —which is the source of the varnishlike sealant that coats the outer surface of the wall.

The main elements of the bottom surface of the foot are the *sole* and the *frog.* The sole, which is concave, joins the bottom edge of the wall at the *white line.* The white line is a narrow horny strip that is a protective continuation of the quick of the hoof and guides the farrier in placing the nails of the horseshoe—they must be driven outside that line. It is not really white—the inner part of the wall is lighter—but it is clearly distinguishable.

At the heel the wall makes a turn to form the *bars* of the hoof. Between them, separated by the *bar grooves,* is the frog.

The Internal Parts

Within the hoof are the three bones of the foot: roughly half of the *short pastern (second phalanx);* the *coffin bone,* shaped like a miniature hoof; and the *navicular bone,* which fits horizontally in the space between the short pastern and the coffin bone. The rear surface of the navicular bone is layered with smooth cartilage, easing the movement of the *flexor tendon* across and under it.

The *lateral cartilage* wings back from the coffin bone on either side of the   189 foot and contributes to the foot's all-important elasticity. It absorbs shock to the bottom of the foot by spreading on impact. The upper rear edges extend to the heel, above the coronet, and can be felt under the skin.

The other effective shock absorber in the foot is the *digital* or *plantar cushion,* occupying the space between the lateral cartilage wings. It is highly elastic and fibrous.

The sensitive parts of the foot are the layers that cover the bones and elastic parts, and all of them produce some part of the hoof. From the *coronary band* (a term that horsemen use interchangeably with "coronet" but that actually applies to an internal part) all the horny hoof grows. The *sensitive laminae*— delicate leaves of tissue—both produce and interlock with the *horny laminae,* this union holding the wall to the coffin bone and lateral cartilage. It is visible as the white line on the bottom of the hoof. The *sensitive sole,* covering the bottom of the coffin bone, produces the horny sole beneath, and the *sensitive frog,* formed on the undersurface of the plantar cushion, produces the frog.

Blood circulation through the foot is generously supplied and is assisted by the pumping action of the striking and raising of the hoof as the horse moves.

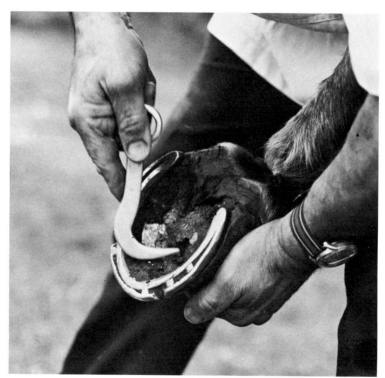

1

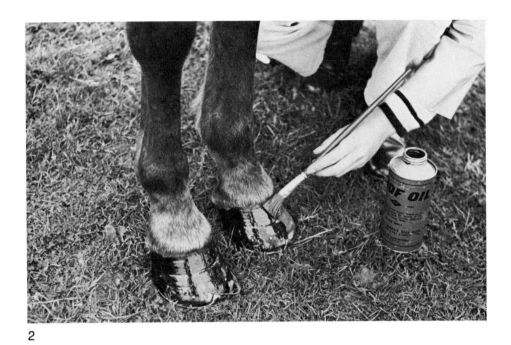

2

A Note on Routine Hoof Care

The routine should include regular trimming by a farrier, regular shoeing, and daily use of the hoof pick to remove irritating pebbles, nails, bits of glass, and so on *(photo 1).* Daily painting of the wall with oil *(photo 2)* to keep it soft and to prevent the formation of cracks may be necessary, depending on the environment.

50. Bruised Sole

The sole, because of its location, is susceptible to bruising. Certain types and breeds of horses are more likely to have the problem than others. For example, the Arab has a very hard sole, whereas the Thoroughbred is much more bruise-prone.

Neglect leading to overgrowth of hoof so that the sole surface becomes flat or convex instead of concave may cause bruised sole. Jumping on stone, or other hard objects, and riding or galloping over stony roads are other causes.

Treatment

Remove the shoes *(photo 1)* and pare out the bruised area so that it is free from pressure *(photo 2);* then poultice and rest for at least a week.

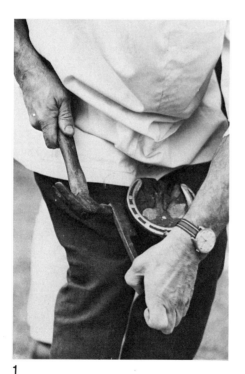

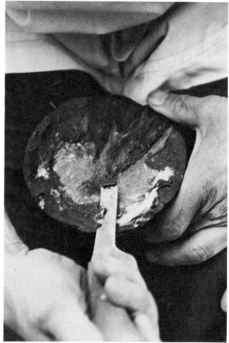

1   2

Thereafter, if you are anxious to get the horse back to work, you can dress the sole with pine tar and place a leather between the shoe and the sole of the horse's foot. Even better than leather is balata belting; this may be difficult to procure, though the broad belts from old belting machines are usually made of this material and, if they are no longer in use on the machine, may be cut up as protective soles when they are required.

Prevention

Simple common sense will prevent bruised sole—regular shoeing and the routine use of the hoof pick, together with the avoidance of stony lanes during exercise or work.

51. Corns

A corn is made by bruising the sole in the sharp angle between the wall and the heel *(photo 1)*. It is often associated with either bad shoeing or the shoe's being left on too long.

Symptoms

Corns cause lameness. Many a so-called "recurring and mysterious lameness" has been proved, on careful searching of the feet, to be the result of a simple corn.

Treatment

This is a job for the veterinarian or the farrier. The shoes have to be removed and the bruised area completely cut out. Thereafter, the shoe can be put on again, but this time with a widened web at the appropriate heel to give protection to the corn area without exerting any pressure.

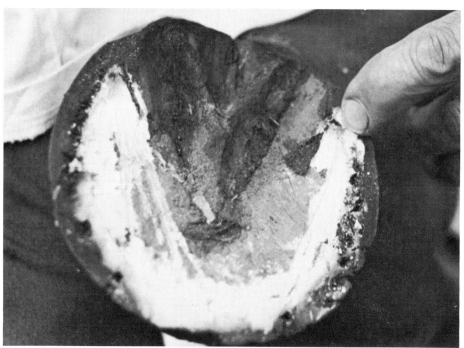

52. Picked-up Nail and Suppurating Feet

When at college, again and again we were told by our professor, "It does not matter where you think a horse is lame; always test the foot." This has proved to be probably the soundest advice of all in horse veterinary practice.

Naturally enough, a horse or a pony is always likely to pick up a nail or to tramp on a sharp piece of metal, stone, glass, or wood—and if any of these foreign objects penetrates the sole to the sensitive structure underneath, subsequent suppuration—pus formation—is a near certainty.

A common place to find a picked-up nail is at or near the point of the frog. The reason for this is simple: the nail gets turned up by the toe; it then slides along the sole until it catches against the frog, where it penetrates.

Symptoms

If the sensitive structures are badly damaged, marked lameness is apparent immediately.

In most cases, however, lameness does not appear for several days. The reason for this is that it is usually four, five, or even six or seven days before the infective material carried in by the nail produces pus and abscess formation. This causes acute pressure on the sensitive areas, and this in turn produces pain, which is often very severe indeed, causing the horse to sweat and paw continually at the ground.

In the early stages, however, the first symptom is usually just pronounced lameness.

When the wall of the affected foot is tapped with a hammer *(photo 1),* the horse will pick the foot up sharply and will often move it up and down and shiver, thus showing clear evidence of pain. The same will happen when the sole is tapped or squeezed between the jaws of a pair of farrier's pincers *(photo 2).* In fact, when searching for the abscess, the veterinarian will often be able to localize the infected area by tapping with the hammer or squeezing with the pincers.

Treatment

Send for your veterinarian immediately. If a nail is present, pull it out but carefully note the spot, to assist the veterinarian upon arrival. Some veterinari-

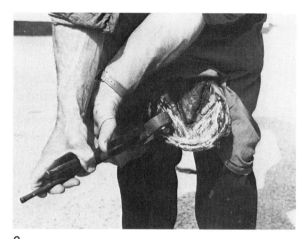

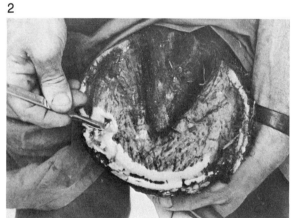

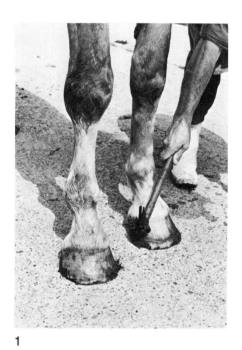

1

2

3

ans will arrange to have a farrier in attendance to remove the shoe and do the cutting out under supervision. Others prefer to do the job on their own.

The main point will be a thorough opening up of the focus of infection to ensure complete drainage *(photo 3).*

If the abscess is not opened up fairly promptly, the pus will take the line of least resistance and the infection will spread either between the sensitive laminae and the sole or between the laminae and the wall. If it follows the latter course, it may burst at the top of the hoof, causing prolonged lameness and the possibility of bone infection. Prompt and efficient drainage is therefore vital.

After the pus has poured out, the cavity should be syringed with antibiotic or antiseptic *(photo 4).*

Subsequently, the foot should be soaked, twice daily in hot water containing antiseptic *(photo 5)* and covered over with a clean sack, or a plastic boot made for this purpose, to prevent the drainage hole from being blocked by dirt.

Another vital treatment is an injection against tetanus. Even if the horse has been innoculated against tetanus, a booster dose of tetanus toxoid is advisable, since puncture wounds in the foot provide the ideal conditions for the growth of tetanus bacteria and also because a wound on the sole of the foot is much more likely to be contaminated by tetanus spores than a wound anywhere else on the body.

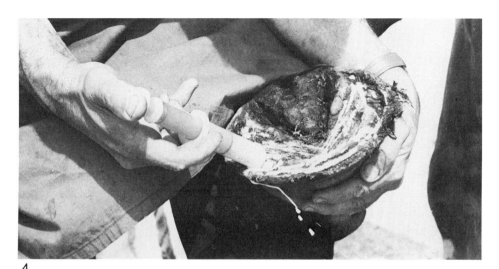

4

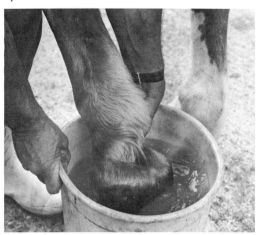

5

53. Thrush

Thrush can be a fungus or a bacterial infection. It involves the frog and is caused by unsanitary conditions—stalls that are not regularly cleaned, for example, or feet that are in poor condition.

Symptoms

In thrush, a dark, foul-smelling discharge *(photo 1)* comes from the cleft between the frog and the sole. If the condition is neglected, it destroys the horn of the frog and may extend into deeper tissues and be quite serious.

Treatment

Clean out the hoof well, particularly around the frog, and treat with a chemical or chemo sterilant, such as iodine, formaldehyde, or copper sulfate. Treat only the infected area around the frog so as not to dry out the whole sole. It may be necessary to trim away the affected portions of the frog. The problem usually responds readily to treatment if the conditions that caused it are corrected, so make sure the stall is kept clean and dry.

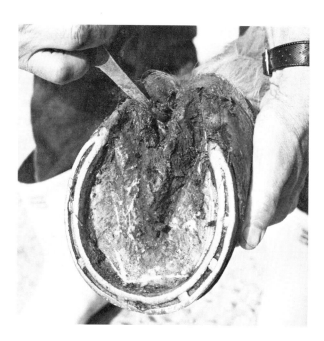

54. Cracked Hooves

Under unfavorable conditions the hoof wall may develop cracks. Cracks follow the "grain" of the horn and vary in severity. Cracks near the ground are commonly called grass cracks, but when a crack extends upward until it reaches the coronet it is called a sand crack *(photo 1)*.

When cracks appear in the hoof wall they usually indicate neglect of the feet. They are most commonly found in the feet of unshod horses, whose hooves have been deprived of regular expert trimming. Prolonged lack of exposure to moisture may cause hooves to become dry and brittle, thus more susceptible to cracking.

Treatment

A notch may be cut in the hoof wall at the lower end of the crack, removing weight from the defective area and decreasing the tendency of the crack to widen. Simple grass cracks will eventually disappear during normal hoof growth.

If the crack is deeper or extends dangerously high the horse may be, or become, debilitated by lameness. Do not hesitate to seek help from an expert farrier or veterinarian. He or she may elect to reinforce the area artificially. Full bar shoes are also helpful in stabilizing the injured area.

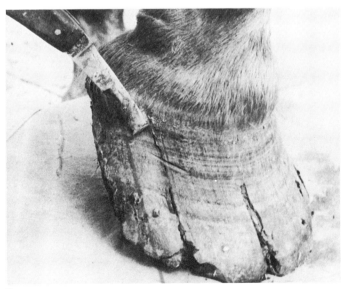

55. Cracked Heels

The term "cracked heel" is a slight misnomer because the condition does not actually occur in the heel but usually in the hollow of the pastern.

Cracked heels *(photo 1)* are usually found in horses or ponies wintered out on soaking wet pastures and mud. They also occur in horses where the legs are washed repeatedly, instead of being brushed, and not dried properly.

Symptoms

The condition starts with scaling and scabbing, which produce nasty, painful cracks. If not treated promptly, the cracks become infected.

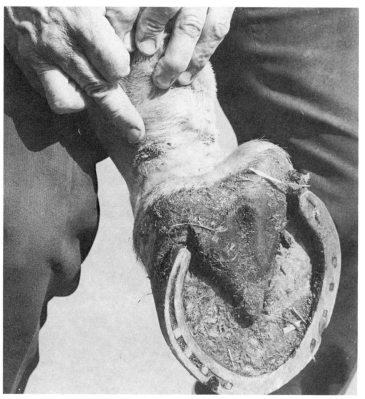

1

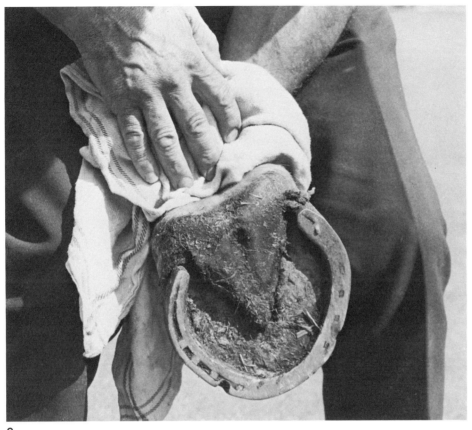

2

The horse may or may not be lame, depending on how long the cracks have been there.

Treatment

Wash well with soap and water to remove all loose matter and then dry *very* thoroughly *(photo 2).*

Apply either Vaseline or any reputable healing and antiseptic ointment, such as thuja ointment or calamine ointment.

Dry powder is contraindicated and should never be used, since it makes the cracks worse. Drying and hardening aerosols also have this adverse effect and should be avoided.

Cortisone creams and ointments tend to slow down healing, but they can also help by limiting formation of excess granulation tissue and thereby the size   201 of the scar. Many veterinarians prescribe cortisone as well as antibiotics as the treatment of choice.

If the horse or pony is lame, he must be rested. If the condition has been caught early and the patient is not lame, confine him to light exercise only during treatment.

Prevention

When the horse or pony is out on wet muddy pastures, a protective smear of Vaseline over the hollow of the pastern at fairly regular intervals will prevent cracking. A twice-weekly dressing should be sufficient.

If the weather and pastures are dry, the protective Vaseline dressing is not necessary.

56. Quittor

In chapter 59 on "Sidebones" there is a simple explanation of lateral cartilages —what they are and where they are situated.

Occasionally, as a result of an injury in the area, part of a lateral cartilage dies. When this happens, a tract of pus travels up toward the hoof head, or coronet, and breaks out, producing a fistula leading directly down to the dead portion of cartilage.

The condition is unmistakable, and invariably the horse is very lame.

Treatment

The only treatment for quittor is surgery, and this should be done by your veterinarian at the earliest possible moment, to avoid involvement of the nearby tendons and bone.

Surgery comprises dissecting down to the damaged cartilage and actually cutting out the dead portion. The resultant wound is then filled with antibiotics or sulfa drugs and bandaged firmly.

The prognosis is quite good provided that the operation is performed without delay.

57. Navicular Disease

Navicular disease is a disease of the navicular bone, a small bone at the back of the foot. It lies across the coffin bone and between it and the second phalanx, acting more or less as a wedge but forming part of the joint. (See chapter 49, *figure 4*).

Along the rear surface of the navicular bone runs the deep flexor tendon. Basically, navicular disease represents a degenerative process involving both the deep flexor tendon and the navicular bone. With time, the navicular bone degenerates, generally on the rear surface, causing hollows and cavities called *lacunae* to appear. This degenerative process of both tendon and bone produces a chronic and persistent pain.

Navicular disease can occur in horses or ponies of any age, but it is most commonly seen in older animals, and often in those that have had a fair amount of percussion on their forefeet during life—for example, through roadwork or

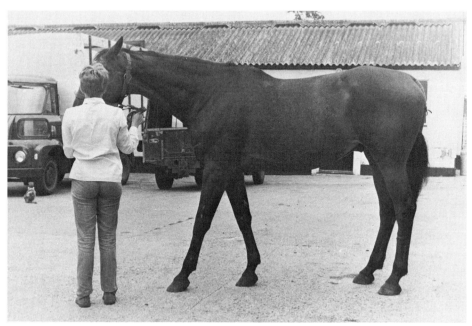

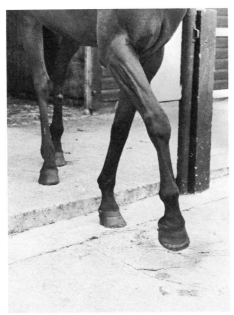

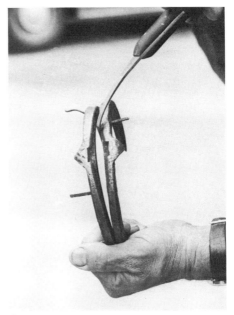

2

3

show jumping. This frequently causes them to "point," standing with one forefoot ahead of the other *(photo 1)*.

It has been my experience that wherever you have a persistent, obscure lameness in the fore end, the most likely cause is navicular disease.

Symptoms

As already stated, any persistent, obscure lameness in the forelegs should always be regarded as a suspect navicular disease. It is much more common in the forefeet; in fact, it is rare in the hind feet. Generally speaking, both forefeet are affected simultaneously. This means that, in the early stages, lameness may not be noticed simply because it is equal in both forelegs.

The typical "navicular gait" is almost diagnostic. The horse "tippy-toes"; that is, he does not extend his forefeet in the normal way but goes with short steps, putting his toes down first in a simple attempt to keep his weight off the heels *(photo 2)*.

An examination of the shoes of a navicular horse will show that the toes are much more worn than the heels *(photo 3)*.

There is also a tendency to stumble, but both the stumbling and the characteristic navicular gait are usually more apparent either when the horse is first brought out of the stable or when the horse is trotted downhill, with the weight being thrown on the front end.

As the disease develops, the hoof first becomes contracted, then what we term "boxy." The walls become more vertical and the heels straight deep, rather like a mule's foot or a donkey's foot.

Diagnosis

Diagnosis can be made on the symptoms with some confidence. The veterinarian may also x-ray the foot *(photo 4)* for supporting evidence, and the x-ray may show lacunae in the bone or a spur at each end. But sometimes the disease will involve only the navicular bursa, and the bone will not be affected until the condition has become chronic.

Before x-raying the foot, however, the veterinarian will probably block the nerves involved in pain of navicular disease by injecting a local anesthetic at a point below the fetlock. The effects of this nerve block will pinpoint the location of the trouble.

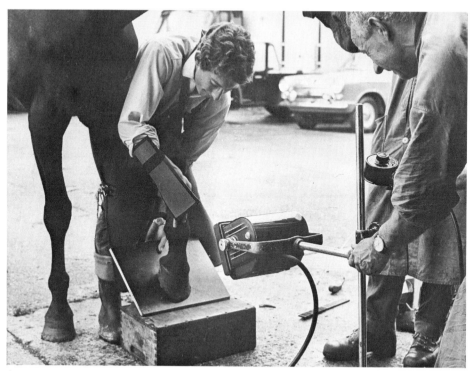

4

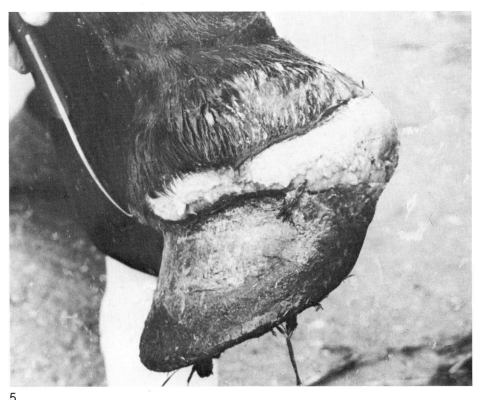

5

Treatment

If the horse is young the disease is detected early, corrective shoes and proper management of exercise may eliminate the symptoms, and the horse will continue to give full usefulness and satisfaction. The same result can be obtained, if necessary, by a neurectomy operation (cutting the nerves that supply the sensation to the area). This is not a cure—there is none—but it removes all pain and thereby stops the lameness.

After neurectomy (often called "denerving"), careful shoeing and daily examination of the feet must be carried out. Should the horse pick up a nail or be pricked when shoeing, infection will set in and it may not be noticed until the sole or wall is extensively underrun *(photo 5)*. This, of course, is what produces the anti-denerving tales of hooves' dropping off after the operation. Obviously neurectomy is not an operation that should be regarded lightly. In my opinion all other modes of therapy should be tried before considering it.

207

58. Founder

Founder, or laminitis, is a condition affecting the feet of horses, usually the forefeet.

The term *laminitis* simply means an inflammation of laminae. The junction between the horny hoof and the coffin bone (which forms the center of the foot) is made by the sensitive laminae (see *figure 4* in chapter 49). The laminae from the hoof and the laminae from the bone dovetail, rather like paper-thin cogs of two minute wheels. When these laminae become inflamed, the condition is laminitis, commonly called founder.

As with all inflammations, swelling occurs—but because of the firm wall of the hoof and sole, there is no room for the swelling and this leads to very acute pain.

Causes

There are several different causes, all producing the same result:

1. Fat ponies that eat too much grass and take very little exercise. It has been my experience that this is by far the commonest cause, especially when the grass contains a high percentage of rich young clover.

2. Feeding too much grain or corn.

3. An allergy.

4. A portion of retained afterbirth or abortion in a mare.

5. Standing for excessively long periods—for instance, when traveling by railroad or ship.

Symptoms

In acute laminitis the temperature rises slightly—one or two degrees—and the pulse rises considerably.

There is very marked lameness, heat around the coronet, and obvious pain when the foot is tapped with a knife handle or a hammer.

The lameness is in the two front feet; when the horse is asked to move, he arches his back, stretches his head out in front of him, and pushes his hind legs underneath in an attempt to take the weight off the forefeet *(photos 1 and 2).*

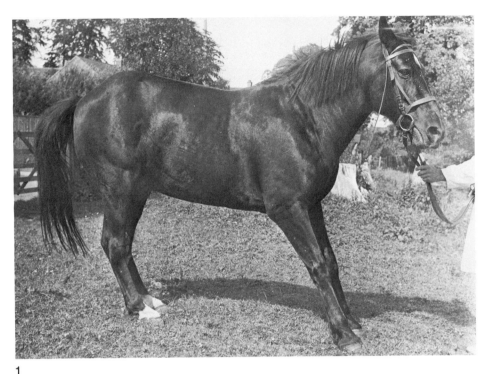

1

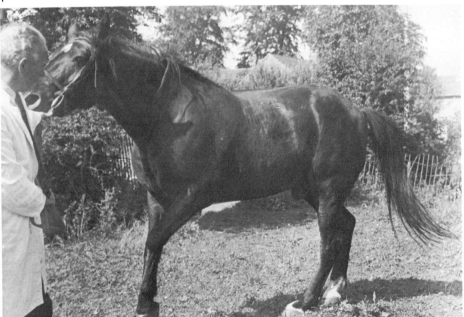

2

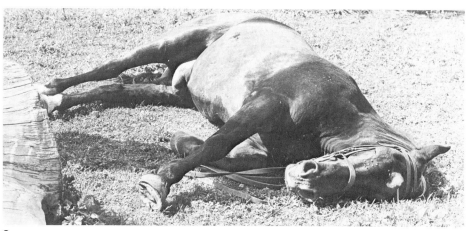

3

He has difficulty in lying down and in getting up—so when he does go down, he will lie, often flat out on his side, for abnormally long periods *(photo 3)*.

If the acute inflammation is prolonged for any length of time, the laminae between the horn and the bone become detached. The weight of the horse then causes the coffin bone to sink downward so that the sole becomes flat instead of concave, or it may even become convex and press on the ground *(photo 4)*.

Also, with the bone sinking, the horny hoof, instead of being straight from the coronary band to the sole's surface, becomes concave and deep ridges appear around the hoof *(photo 5)*.

All this produces what is recognized as *chronic* laminitis.

Treatment

Acute laminitis is an emergency and should be treated quickly. Prompt treatment can reduce the inflammation rapidly and do much to prevent the "dropped sole." So it is vitally important to call the veterinarian whenever this disease is suspected.

The cause must be ascertained and rectified at once. For example, if the laminitis results from overfeeding, the horse must be given the lightest possible diet.

If the horse or pony is on pasture, he should be housed in a spacious box stall, well bedded down with sphagnum moss or sawdust, and ample fresh drinking water should be provided.

Local treatment, such as cold hosing from the fetlocks downward three or four times a day *(photo 6),* or standing the horse in a cold running brook

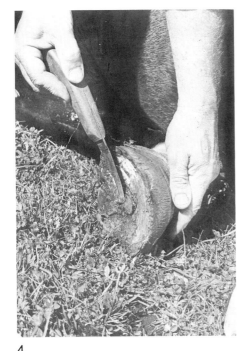

4

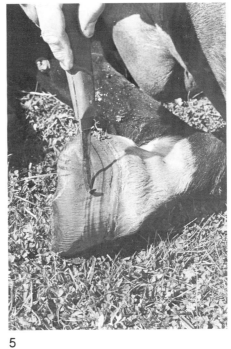

5

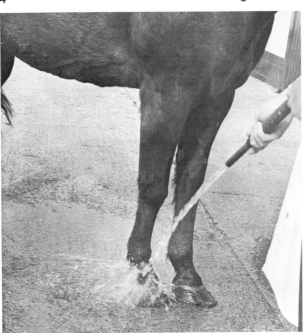

6

for several half-hour periods during the day, can be very helpful. A cold, wet mud poultice, kept cold and wet by pouring water over it, can also be used.

Chronic cases require special (broad-webbed seated out) surgical shoes which should be made under veterinary supervision and fitted hot; they should be renewed at least once a month.

Prevention

Preventing founder is far better than having to treat it and is quite simple. Avoid all the likely causes—if a mare holds her afterbirth, have her attended to at once. Never overfeed, and do not leave fat ponies to gorge themselves on rich pastures.

59. Sidebones

Once again some knowledge of simple anatomy is required to understand exactly what a sidebone is.

On each side of the coffin bone (the lowest bone of the foot), there is a wing of cartilage called the lateral cartilage (see *figure 1*).

Frequently in heavy horses, but rarely in the lighter breeds and ponies, this cartilage changes into bone. When this happens, the resultant hard lump of bone is called a sidebone.

In heavy horses the ossification often occurs spontaneously for no apparent reason, but in light horses or ponies the cause is usually an injury of some sort.

Symptoms

Lameness is often negligible or completely absent. The hard bone formation can be felt by attempting to flex the cartilage or bend it inward *(photo 1)*. Occasionally, it is a chronic source of problems.

Treatment

Usually a shoeing problem is present, such as foot imbalance. The treatment, then, is a correction of such an imbalance. The addition of pads to absorb concussion is also helpful.

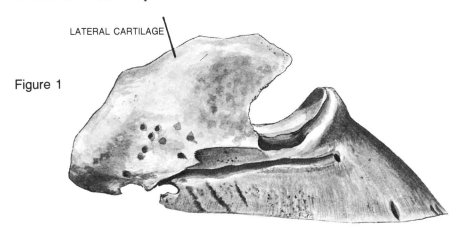

LATERAL CARTILAGE

Figure 1

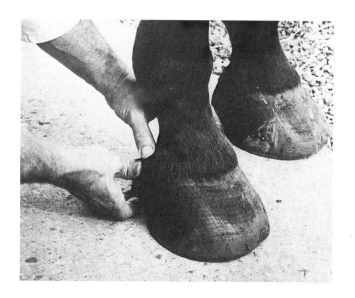

Are Sidebones an Unsoundness?

Yes, although they are often not significant. Radiographs (x-rays) would be helpful prior to purchase in suspected cases.

Prognosis

Prognosis varies, but generally the condition is not a serious one.

214

60. Seedy Toe

Seedy toe is a separation of the wall of the hoof from the sensitive laminae, or quick *(photo 1)*.

A seedy toe can start with a slight crack or injury between the sole and the wall. Dirt may gradually work into the cavity, eventually producing a seedy toe.

The most common cause, however, is foot neglect. In fact, seedy toe could be said to be a frequent complication of lack of foot care. What happens is that the overgrown wall is pushed away from the soft tissues by the weight of the horse. Subsequently, small stones or dirt pack in and enlarge the space. Occasionally abscesses develop, further complicating the picture (see chapter 52).

Seedy toe often accompanies chronic laminitis (see chapter 58).

Symptoms

The first sign of seedy toe is usually lameness. Examination of the foot will reveal a dead space filled with debris between the sole and the wall.

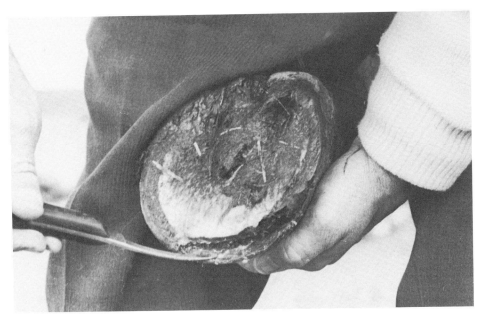

1

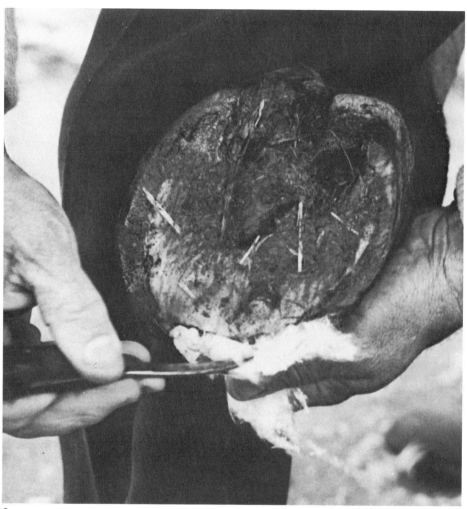

2

Treatment

Remove all dirt and grit, and hollow out the seedy toe to its full extent. Clip and dress the foot. This is a job for your veterinarian or farrier.

Pack the cavity with tar and tow, or with absorbent cotton soaked in an oily suspension of antibiotic *(photo 2),* and shoe with a broad-webbed shoe with the web covering the packed cavity.

Some veterinarians recommend blistering the coronary band to stimulate the growth of new horn, but it is my opinion that this is unnecessary, especially if the foot is subsequently looked after carefully and shod regularly.

INDEX

Index

Italicized page numbers indicate photographs or drawings

223